Patient-Centered Assisted Reproduction

T0201375

Patient-Centered Assisted Reproduction

How to Integrate Exceptional Care with Cutting-Edge Technology

Edited by

Alice D Domar
Boston IVF, Waltham, MA

Denny Sakkas
Boston IVF, Waltham, MA

Thomas L Toth
Boston IVF, Waltham, MA

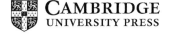
CAMBRIDGE
UNIVERSITY PRESS

CAMBRIDGE
UNIVERSITY PRESS

University Printing House, Cambridge CB2 8BS, United Kingdom

One Liberty Plaza, 20th Floor, New York, NY 10006, USA

477 Williamstown Road, Port Melbourne, VIC 3207, Australia

314–321, 3rd Floor, Plot 3, Splendor Forum, Jasola District Centre, New Delhi – 110025, India

79 Anson Road, #06–04/06, Singapore 079906

Cambridge University Press is part of the University of Cambridge.

It furthers the University's mission by disseminating knowledge in the pursuit of education, learning, and research at the highest international levels of excellence.

www.cambridge.org
Information on this title: www.cambridge.org/9781108796774
DOI: 10.1017/9781108859486

© Alice D Domar, Denny Sakkas, and Thomas L Toth 2020

This publication is in copyright. Subject to statutory exception and to the provisions of relevant collective licensing agreements, no reproduction of any part may take place without the written permission of Cambridge University Press.

First published 2020

Printed in the United Kingdom by TJ International Ltd. Padstow Cornwall

A catalogue record for this publication is available from the British Library.

ISBN 978-1-108-79677-4 Paperback

Cambridge University Press has no responsibility for the persistence or accuracy of URLs for external or third-party internet websites referred to in this publication and does not guarantee that any content on such websites is, or will remain, accurate or appropriate.

....

Every effort has been made in preparing this book to provide accurate and up-to-date information that is in accord with accepted standards and practice at the time of publication. Although case histories are drawn from actual cases, every effort has been made to disguise the identities of the individuals involved. Nevertheless, the authors, editors, and publishers can make no warranties that the information contained herein is totally free from error, not least because clinical standards are constantly changing through research and regulation. The authors, editors, and publishers therefore disclaim all liability for direct or consequential damages resulting from the use of material contained in this book. Readers are strongly advised to pay careful attention to information provided by the manufacturer of any drugs or equipment that they plan to use.

Contents

Contributors

Antonio Capalbo PhD
IGENOMIX, Marostica, Italy and
IGENOMIX, Parque Tecnologico Paterna,
Valencia, Spain

Lindsay Childress-Beatty JD PhD
Office of Ethics, American Psychological
Association, Washington, DC, USA

Monica Clemente PhD
IGENOMIX, Parque Tecnologico Paterna,
Valencia, Spain

Thomas M D'Hooghe MD PhD
Global Medical Affairs Fertility, Research
and Development, Merck Biopharma
KGaA, Darmstadt, Germany and
Department of Development and
Regeneration, Biomedical Sciences Group,
KU Leuven (University of Leuven),
Leuven, Belgium

Alice D Domar PhD
Domar Centers for Mind/Body Health,
Boston IVF, Beth Israel Deaconess
Medical Center, Harvard Medical
School, USA

Kevin Doody MD
Center for Assisted Reproduction,
Bedford, TX, USA

Kaitlin Doody MD
University of Texas Southwestern Medical
Center, Dallas, TX, USA

Sofia Gameiro PhD
Cardiff Fertility Studies Research Group,
Cardiff University, Cardiff, UK

David K Gardner DPhil
School of BioSciences, University of
Melbourne, and Melbourne IVF,
Melbourne, Australia

Jan Gerris MD PhD
University Women's Clinic, Ghent
University Hospital, Ghent, Belgium

Elizabeth Grill PsyD
The Ronald O. Perelman and Claudia
Cohen Center for Reproductive Medicine,
Weill Cornell Medical College, New York,
NY, USA

Karin Hammarberg RN PhD
Jean Hailes Research Unit, School of
Public Health & Preventive Medicine,
Monash University, Melbourne, Victoria,
Australia

Sarah R Holley PhD
Clinical Psychology, San Francisco State
University, San Francisco, CA, USA

Colin M Howles PhD
Department of Biomedical Sciences,
University of Edinburgh, UK and
ARIES Consulting, Geneva, Switzerland

Marcia Inhorn PhD
Department of Anthropology, Yale
University, New Haven, CT, USA

Emily Koert PhD
Department of Educational &
Counselling Psychology, University of
British Columbia, Vancouver, BC,
Canada

Angela Q Leung MD
Boston IVF, Beth Israel Deaconess,
Medical Center, Harvard Medical School,
Boston, MA, USA

Jeroen Luyten PhD
Leuven Institute for Healthcare Policy,
Department of Public Health and Primary
Care, KU Leuven, Belgium

Gritt Marie Hviid Malling MSc
Department of Public Health, University of Copenhagen, Copenhagen, Denmark

Lauri A Pasch PhD
Department of Psychiatry, University of California, San Francisco, CA, USA

Pasquale Patrizio MD MBE HCLD
Yale Fertility Center, Department of Obstetrics, Gynecology and Reproductive Sciences, New Haven, CT, USA

Maurizio Poli DPhil
IGENOMIX, Marostica, Italy

Carmen Rubio PhD
IGENOMIX, Parque Tecnologico Paterna, Valencia, Spain

Denny Sakkas PhD
Boston IVF, Waltham, MA, USA

Lone Schmidt DMSci PhD MD
Department of Public Health, University of Copenhagen, Copenhagen, Denmark

Carlos Simon MD PhD
IGENOMIX, Parque Tecnologico Paterna, Valencia, Spain

Thomas L Toth MD
Boston IVF, Beth Israel Deaconess, Medical Center, Harvard Medical School, Boston, MA, USA

Evelyn Verbeke PhD candidate
Leuven Institute for Healthcare Policy, Department of Public Health and Primary Care, KU Leuven, Belgium

Introduction

Alice D Domar, Denny Sakkas, and Thomas L Toth

Just before Lesley Brown naturally ovulated on November 9, 1977, she underwent laparoscopic surgery to aspirate the fluid in her left ovary, which contained a single egg. It was fertilized with the sperm of Lesley's husband, John. Three days later, the resulting embryo contained eight cells and was transferred into Lesley's uterus. On July 25, 1978, history was made with the arrival of the first baby conceived via in vitro fertilization (IVF).

Unlike today, Lesley did not take gonadotropins or antagonist medication, she did not meet with a mental health professional who specialized in fertility counseling, neither she nor John underwent genetic testing, nor was the embryo tested for genetic abnormalities, the success rate prior to Louise's conception was zero (out of more than 300 attempts), there was no technology available for Lesley or John to communicate with their medical team other than the telephone, Lesley was not offered the option to freeze any surplus embryos or eggs (if there had been any), and the couple was not crippled by debt from their attempts. In addition, previously Lesley had had to undergo unsuccessful salpingostomies; the only treatment available for her.

In the next decade or more, although oocyte retrievals would be accomplished via a vaginal ultrasound probe, women had to cope with at least daily intramuscular injections of not only progesterone in oil during the luteal phase but also gonadotropins during the follicular phase. These medications came in glass vials and patients had to break the vials and then mix the contents prior to injection. Women faced a significant risk of ovarian hyperstimulation syndrome (OHSS) with resulting hospitalization. Perilous, multiple embryo transfers (ETs) were performed to try and improve pregnancy rates but at the detriment of risking multiple births leading to complication for mother and child(ren). Transfers were done without ultrasound guidance, there were no significant options for severe male factor (SMF), treatment was only offered to married heterosexual couples, and pregnancy rates were slow to increase.

Fast forward another 30-plus years and the technology, pharmacology, psychology, ethics, and options available to individuals and couples today are dazzling. Most patients who undergo assisted reproductive technology (ART) have close to a 50% chance of delivering a healthy baby, with many of them having the option to freeze eggs, sperm, embryos, and blastocysts. Embryos are grown in the laboratory to day five when biopsy is easily accomplished. This technology can now be extended not only to infertile individuals and couples but also to those who are known carriers of genetic diseases to eliminate the risk of passing along these genetic abnormalities. Male factor can be effortlessly compensated for with intracytoplasmic sperm injection (ICSI), recombinant gonadotropins come premixed and measured and are delivered subcutaneously, and family-building options are routinely offered to those not a part of a heterosexual couple, including single women and men. Gay men can achieve genetic parenthood with egg donation and gestational surrogacy, gay women can use sperm donation, and lesbian couples can share in the biological creation of their children through partner-assisted

1

reproduction. In addition, women can now freeze their eggs in an effort to counter the negative impact of ageing on oocyte quality.

However, all these advancements can come at a cost. Health-care professionals in the reproductive medicine field have to balance the time commitment required to stay current with the most recent treatment advances while offering the best in patient care. This can be challenging to anyone.

The goal of this book is to provide physicians, nurses, embryologists, technicians, mental health professionals, and administrators with the information they need to achieve that balance, as well as to have a glimpse into the future.

In the following chapters, readers will be introduced to the most cutting-edge available options such as predictive genetic modeling, new medication delivery systems, personalized medicine as applied to the environment for each embryo, and an end of the necessity for numerous clinic visits for monitoring. And in what will truly represent the ART field of the future is a model for patient-centered care, achieved via integrative care, new methods of patient communication such as social media and digital applications, fertility preservation (FP), a consideration of patient options leading to ethical quandaries, approaches to lessen the psychological impact of treatment that can increase patient and nursing retention, and discussions on how to lessen the financial impact on patients and how to provide broader access for infertility patients through both public avenues and innovative technologies.

Finally, the last chapter will put it all together, leading the reader through the cycle of the future: what will be offered to each individual from a technical, pharmaceutical, psychological, and clinic process perspective, seen from the eyes of a couple undergoing an ART cycle who could well be your patients to be. And can become parents to be.

Access to Infertility Care

Kevin Doody and Kaitlin Doody

ART has made great advancements in the last several decades. From 3D sonographic imaging to assess for mullerian anomalies, to new medications and treatment protocols, the science of infertility treatment is constantly evolving. As technology improves, there continues to be a rising demand for fertility services. In fact, over eight million children worldwide have been born as a consequence of ART. However, despite these advancements, ART is available to only a small portion of the affected population. Numerous barriers prohibit many couples from accessing the services required to create a family. Economic cost is one of the most common obstacles that a patient will cite. However, it is important to consider the geographic, cultural, and psychological obstacles the infertile couple or individual may also face.

It has been estimated that 11% of women of reproductive age in the United States experience difficulties with infertility. Not all women experiencing infertility seek care with fertility specialists. In 2009 it was estimated that only about a quarter of ART needs were being met in the United States[1]. Unfortunately, there is little research exploring the limited utilization of fertility resources both in the United States and worldwide. The majority of the available studies have focused primarily on the affordability factor. However, accessibility can be heavily influenced by other social factors, such as geography, race, gender identity, and sexuality. There are likely countless other confounding factors also contributing to this disparity. It is important to recognize that there are distinct groups, both in the United States and internationally, that are unable to access the care they may need to create a family.

Despite healthcare mandates and improvement in ART technology, there has been little change in the number and demographic of people who undergo evaluation and receive fertility treatments. This chapter will present the different barriers to care and recent groundbreaking initiatives to overcome these obstacles.

Financial Barriers

Numerous studies have shown one of the most common barriers to accessing fertility care is the cost of treatment. At the time this chapter was written, the United States has some of the most expensive ART in the world. The average cost of a single IVF cycle in the United States in 2014 was $12 400 USD. That same year the average cost of a cycle in Europe was $5000 USD[2]. Infertility care is often excluded from health insurance plans in the United States; therefore, most patients are required to pay out of pocket for the majority of their treatments. The cost of an IVF cycle can be prohibitive and limits the treatment options available to those who require infertility services. Even non-IVF treatments, such as intrauterine insemination (IUI), may be cost-prohibitive as the required hormonal medications alone can cost several thousand dollars[3].

Decreased patient costs have been shown to increase the utilization rates of fertility services. These costs are different around the world due to the variety of healthcare systems. Comparative analysis of different countries has demonstrated a correlation between affordability of ART and utilization rates. Scandinavian countries have some of the most comprehensive government funding for infertility treatment. These countries show significantly higher rates of utilization despite rates of infertility comparable to the United States[4]. It is suspected that, by alleviating some of the financial burden from the individual patient, more people are willing to seek treatment.

State-mandated insurance coverage for IVF has been proposed and implemented in several states as a way to increase access to care within the United States. At the time of publishing, there are 16 states with some form of infertility insurance coverage laws. The degree of coverage and requirements for eligibility vary widely by state. Similar to what has been observed comparing different countries, studies within the United States have demonstrated higher utilization rates of infertility treatment in states with comprehensive mandates compared to those without. While the larger political debate surrounding government-mandated insurance is beyond the scope of this chapter, these studies highlight that more affordable treatment is correlated with increased access to care and utilization. There may be other unexpected benefits to decreasing patient costs. Some studies have noted a possible association with fewer embryos transferred per cycle in states with mandated insurance coverage and countries with more affordable care. It is suspected that couples may feel less pressured to transfer more than one embryo in a single cycle if the financial burden is lifted[5,6].

Drivers of High Cost of Fertility Treatment

IVF has evolved to be a complex process, which requires an expensive infrastructure. The cost to the patient comes not only from the medications and procedures but also the general overhead cost of running a fertility clinic. The process of stimulating the ovaries to prepare for egg retrieval generally involves many visits for hormonal testing and ultrasound evaluations of the ovary. Patients are often required to learn how to self-inject hormonal medications. Not only do these medications come at a high cost to the patients (often thousands of dollars per cycle), but the complexity of the medication schedules also requires the clinics to provide teaching on how to administer appropriately. As much of the stimulation process relies on the patient's ability to properly give these medications at home, the clinic needs highly trained staff to communicate results and instructions effectively.

IVF facilities and the required embryology laboratories are costly, due to both the high infrastructure cost and the requirement for constant monitoring for safe storage of oocytes and embryos. The proper environment for managing and storing human embryos must be highly controlled. Human embryos lack organs such as lungs, kidneys, or livers to filter or remove toxins. Ambient air contains volatile organic compounds (VOCs) that impede embryonic development. Therefore, good IVF laboratories will have sophisticated heating, ventilation, and air conditioning systems designed to remove not only particles, but also these VOCs. Specialized incubators are required to provide the appropriate temperature, low oxygen, and high carbon dioxide concentrations. Because these are complex electromechanical devices, they need quality control checks each day. Achieving good quality control requires special instruments to undergo periodic calibration. Additionally, the incubators and embryo storage units can fail completely. Because this equipment houses something as precious as human embryos, the devices must be monitored at all times with a reliable alarm system.

Geographic Barriers

Physical access to infertility care is another potential obstacle to obtaining treatment. While many general obstetrics-gynecology practitioners may provide basic medical and surgical therapies to treat infertility, many patients require specific services provided only by fertility clinics. This may include diagnostic procedures, such as hysteroscopies and hysterosalpingograms, or treatment therapies such as IVF, ICSI, and preimplantation genetic testing (PGT). The evaluation and treatment course may span several months, requiring frequent visits for monitoring and procedures.

The United States lacks adequate distribution of infertility providers. There are approximately 1300 board-certified reproductive endocrinologists practicing in the United States, with about 50 graduating from fellowship programs every year. There are many women across the United States who may not live in an area that provides fertility treatment. Reproductive endocrinologists are primarily centered in dense urban areas. Geographic analysis has identified that IVF clinics are generally not available in cities with a population less than 250 000. This leaves those living in more rural areas without easily accessible resources. It has been estimated that 18 million women of reproductive age live in regions without access to ART providers, while another seven million live in a region with only a single ART provider[7]. While few patients may have the ability to travel great distances to reach appropriately trained providers, many do not have the resources required to seek out care.

Even those who live in close proximity to an IVF clinic may struggle with the time required for treatments. Many individualized protocols within the United States require multiple clinic visits for sonographic and laboratory hormone monitoring for a single cycle. Patients may face difficulty getting the required time off work as many people prefer to keep infertility treatments a private matter.

Social and Cultural Barriers

Given social and economic factors are often closely intertwined, it appears improvement in access to care is affected by more than decreasing cost. Similar rates of infertility are found among women of all races, socioeconomic status, and education levels. A study in 2005 surveyed women in the state of Massachusetts who underwent evaluation of infertility and found that there were significant educational and racial disparities. Despite the implementation of a broad mandate of six IVF cycles covered per pregnancy, African-American and Hispanic women, as well as those with less than a high-school degree, were underrepresented among those who were receiving treatment[8].

Different cultures may have stigmas surrounding the concept of infertility and may not be aware of the appropriate time to seek help. Nor may they know how to seek assistance. In many developing countries, particularly sub-Saharan Africa and South Asia, misinformation regarding infertility can cause significant social consequences for women. Some cultures do not recognize male factor infertility and, as a consequence, women are often blamed and even ostracized for the inability to conceive a child. The social repercussions of childlessness are often overlooked as these resource-poor countries are battling numerous health crises.

Members of the lesbian, gay, bisexual, transgender, queer/questioning (LGBTQ) community may encounter barriers to accessing treatment that heterosexual couples would not experience. Same-sex couples often experience greater costs for treatment, whether that be for gamete donation or a gestational surrogate. Same-sex couples, transgender patients, and unmarried persons may be denied treatment by clinics. While many states provide protection for these individuals, not all states have such laws to prevent discrimination. The American Society for Reproductive Medicine (ASRM) has published strong ethics committee opinion statements emphasizing the responsibility of fertility providers to offer evaluation and treatment to all people of the previously mentioned groups[9,10].

Psychological

It is important to recognize the emotional impact that the inability to conceive spontaneously may have on women as well as their partners. There are some studies regarding the psychological consequences of the diagnosis of infertility and fertility treatments, but information on how this impacts access to care is limited. One study reported that depressed women are significantly less likely to initiate ART treatment[11], and another study[12] demonstrated that depression in the female partner was the greatest predictor of treatment termination. Numerous studies have shown that the emotional burden of care is the most commonly cited reason for insured women to drop out of treatment. In addition, many patients undergoing infertility treatment may also have concurrent psychiatric diagnoses, caused or exacerbated by the experience of infertility. A recent 2015 study demonstrated an increased prevalence of major depressive disorder (MDD) in both men and women undergoing infertility treatment compared to the general population. It found 39% of women and 15% of men met criteria for MDD at some point during the period of treatment. This is compared to 8% of women and 5% of men in the general population of the United States. The study also highlighted that individuals with a history of MDD were at an even greater risk of developing MDD during infertility treatment likely due to the increased psychological stress[13]. It is important for a provider to recognize that psychological symptoms can present during the treatment process and possibly hinder a patient's motivation or desire to complete the evaluation or treatment process. This can have significant impact on a patient's relationships and ability to function in their day-to-day life. Couples pursuing infertility evaluation may hide their treatment process from their friends and family due to feelings of guilt and shame[14]. It is important for a provider to recognize early signs and symptoms of anxiety or depression. It may be necessary for a provider to screen high-risk patients for psychological symptoms, and then provide appropriate resources and/or referral to a behavioral health provider[15].

Initiatives to Increase Access to Care

It is clear that trying to tackle the problem of limited access to infertility care will not be achieved with a single solution given the numerous social and economic aspects. Infertility and childlessness are understudied aspects of family planning, which can have significant social repercussions in both the developed and underdeveloped world. While persons living in both developed and developing countries may experience similar psychological stressors as discussed earlier in this chapter, those living in resource-poor countries often have added social effects. Women are often blamed, though they may not be the affected partner. These women often become marginalized and stigmatized within their community. As expected, fertility treatment is especially cost-prohibitive in these countries and leaves those affected with limited options. There are organizations and companies around the world that are working to find solutions.

Over the last few years, the ASRM has attempted to highlight the unmet needs in infertility care both in the United States and globally. In 2015, the ASRM published an ethics committee opinion outlining disparities in access to care, stating the "creation of a family is a basic human right." The goal of the published statement was to encourage researchers to further explore barriers to care and opportunities for improvement. In September of the same year, the ASRM held the Access to Care Summit to develop strategies to expand care both in the United States and abroad. During the summit it was recognized that infertility was not considered a disease in the greater medical community or government, therefore minimizing its impact on quality of life. In 2017, the ASRM worked with the American Medical Association (AMA) to pass a resolution designating infertility as a disease. This statement was consistent with the World Health Organization's (WHO) stance since 2009.

While the conversation around increasing access to care has been evolving and growing in the last several years, there have been proponents since the creation of IVF. RESOLVE: The National Infertility Association is a patient advocacy organization, which was established in 1974. It works to bring awareness of large-scale fertility issues to patients, the medical community, and politicians. RESOLVE created an annual advocacy day, which brings members of the infertility community, patients, and medical providers to Washington DC to speak with politicians to advocate for access to care and improved coverage. In the spring of 2019, the ASRM and RESOLVE announced a partnership to further expand these efforts.

The intravaginal culture (IVC) is a creative solution to low-cost infertility treatment, which has been explored since the 1980s. IVC for the fertilization of eggs and embryos was first discovered as an IVF/embryo culture option in the 1980s when a French embryologist brainstormed to ensure proper care of retrieved eggs and processed sperm following an unanticipated power outage[16]. Ranoux used improvised laboratory materials (vials used for sperm cryo-storage vials wrapped in paraffin film) and placed them in the intended mother's vagina to provide the appropriate temperature environment for fertilization and embryo development. The recognition that fertilization and

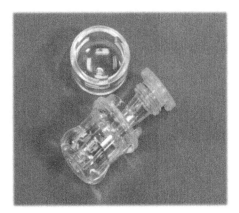

Figure 1.1 INVOcell device

early embryo development was able to be accomplished in an IVC system generated a great deal of enthusiasm. During the 1990s several investigators from many countries reported the use of IVC with improvised devices in conjunction with mild ovarian stimulation or natural cycles with success. Success varied and ultimately the limitations associated with the use of improvised devices prevented widespread adoption. These limitations included occasional bacterial contamination of the media and a negative impact of air bubbles that were difficult to avoid and detect during the loading of gametes. A device specifically designed for IVC (the INVOcell device, Figure 1.1) was approved by the United States Food and Drug Administration (FDA) in 2015. This device was designed to prevent the limitations encountered with the improvised devices. By housing the gametes within the patient's vagina, an ideal environment (temperature, pH, etc.) is created without requiring a sophisticated embryology laboratory. The need for back-up power, clean air systems, alarms, and so on is avoided.

A randomized-prospective open-label trial was performed in 2014 to compare the IVC device with traditional IVF with extended embryo culture. The results demonstrated similar quality embryos at the time of transfer with comparable live birth rates with both incubation systems. The IVC device not only decreases the cost through use of the device itself but also has a streamlined protocol, which limits patient visits and laboratory testing. The previously mentioned trial used a strict medication protocol with human menopausal gonadotropin in a fixed gonadotropin-releasing hormone cycle, which was calculated based on the patient's anti-Müllerian hormone (AMH) and body mass index (BMI). There was only one monitoring ultrasound that was performed during stimulation. By decreasing medication costs and clinic visits, the device and treatment protocol helps to combat both the cost and geographic barriers that many patients face[17].

The Walking Egg project is a nonprofit organization, which was created in 2010 with the goal of bringing together different fields to discuss and promote access to fertility care in especially resource-poor areas. The organization works with the WHO and the European Society for Human Reproduction and Embryology (ESHRE) to bring medical experts, economists, political scientists, and patients together to study and advocate for affordable and accessible infertility treatment worldwide. Many international organizations recognize the importance of primary prevention of infertility by public health education and awareness. This includes safe sex practices, given sexually transmitted infections are a primary cause of male and female infertility worldwide. However, few organizations have focused resources on the treatment of infertility in these countries. The Walking Egg project is one of the first organizations to focus on improving access to treatment. By establishing "one-stop clinics" their goal is to increase access, affordability, and utilization of ART services in resource-poor countries. Their primary focus is on standardized and low-cost IVF and non-IVF protocols, including IUI with natural cycles and low dose stimulation[18,19].

The Walking Egg project has also created a simplified closed culture system in an attempt to reduce overall IVF costs. Their method involved the combination of citric acid and sodium bicarbonate to generate a pH and atmospheric conditions similar to that of traditional IVF incubators. The oocytes and spermatozoa are initially placed within fertilization tubes and then transferred to a glass vacutainer containing the culture medium. The containers are then stored in a warm water bath. Different than the INVOcell protocol, this method requires much of the continuous monitoring that traditional IVF requires. Given that human embryos are extremely sensitive to changes in the environment, this method requires continuous monitoring of water temperature, as well as a constant and reliable energy source to supply heat to the water bath[20].

The AneVivo device is another recent attempt to challenge traditional IVF. Similar to the INVOcell device, it allows for natural regulation of the environment as fertilization takes place within the woman's body. However, this device is more invasive as one end is placed through the cervix into the intrauterine cavity, while the other end rests within the vagina. The spermatozoa and oocytes are housed within a porous chamber within the end in the intrauterine cavity. After fertilization and development of the embryos, the device is removed and then the embryos are transferred in the traditional fashion. However, there is little data at the time of writing as to the safety and efficacy of this device.

Conclusion

The issue of limited access to ART care is complex and multifaceted. Decreasing economic costs through increased coverage and simplifying ART practices will likely cause significant impact on accessibility. However, it is essential to consider and advocate for subgroups within the population, both in the United States and abroad, who face considerable social barriers. It will take a combination of initiatives, both political and scientific, to expand the population of people able to access the care to expand their families.

References

1. Disparities in Access to Effective Treatment for Infertility in the United States: An Ethics Committee Opinion. *Fertil Steril.* 2015; 104(5): 1104–10.

2. The Funding of IVF Treatment. ESHRE Fact Sheets 4. January 2017.

3. Chambers, et al. The Economic Impact of Assisted Reproductive Technology: A Review of Selected Developed Countries. *Fertil Steril.* 2009; 91(6): 2281–94.

4. Chambers, et al. The Impact of Consumer Affordability on Access to Assisted Reproductive Technologies and Embryo Transfer Practices: An International Analysis. *Fertil Steril.* 2014; 101(1): 191–8.

5. Jain T, Harlow BL, Hornstein MD. Insurance Coverage and Outcomes of in Vitro Fertilization. *N Engl J Med.* 2002; 347 (9):661–6.

6. Crawford S Assisted Reproductive Technology Use, Embryo Transfer Practices, and Birth Outcomes After Infertility Insurance Mandates: New Jersey and Connecticut. *Fertil Steril.* 2016; 105(2): 347–55.

7. Harris JA. Geographic Access to Assisted Reproductive Technology Health Care in the United States: A Population-Based Cross-Sectional Study. *Fertil Steril.* 2017; 107(4): 1023–7.

8. Jain et al. Disparities in Access to Infertility Services in a State with Mandated Insurance Coverage. *Fertil Steril.* 2005; 84(1): 221–3.

9. Ethics Committee of the American Society for Reproductive Medicine. Access to Fertility Treatment by Gays, Lesbians, and Unmarried Persons: A Committee Opinion. *Fertil Steril.* 2013; 100(6): 1524–7.

10. Ethics Committee of the American Society for Reproductive Medicine. Access to Fertility Services by Transgender Persons: An Ethics Committee Opinion. *Fertil Steril.* 2015; 104(5): 1111–15.

11. Crawford NM, et al. Infertile Women Who Screen Positive for Depression Are Less Likely to Initiate Fertility Treatments. *Hum Reprod.* 2017; 32(3): 582–7.

12. Pedro J, et al. Couples' Discontinuation of Fertility Treatments: A Longitudinal Study on Demographic, Biomedical, and Psychosocial Risk Factors. *J Assist Reprod Genet.* 2017; 34(2): 217–24.

13. Holley, et al. Prevalence and Predictors of Major Depressive Disorder for Fertility Treatment Patients and Their Partners. *Fertil Steril.* 2015; 103(5): 1332–9.

14. Galhardo A. The Impact of Shame and Self-Judgment on Psychopathology in Infertile Patients. *Hum Reprod.* 2011; 26(9): 2408–14.

15. Rich C, Domar, A. Addressing the Emotional Barriers to Access to Reproductive Care. *Fertil Steril.* 2016; 105(5): 1124–7.

16. Ranoux C. A New in Vitro Fertilization Technique: Intravaginal Culture. *Fertil Steril.* 1988; 49(4): 654–7.

17. Doody K. Comparing Blastocyst Quality and Live Birth Rates of Intravaginal Culture Using INVOcell to Traditional in vitro Incubation in a Randomized Open-Label Prospective Controlled Trial. *J Assist Reprod Genet.* 2016; 33: 4495–500.

18. Ombelet W. The Walking Egg Project: Universal Access to Infertility Care – from Dream to Reality. *Facts, Views & Visions in Obgyn.* 2013; 5(2): 161–75.

19. Ombelet W. Is Global Access to Infertility Care Realistic? The Walking Egg Project. *Reprod Biomed Online* 2014. 28(3): 267–72.

20. Van Blerkom J, et al. First Births with a Simplified Culture System for Clinical IVF and Embryo Transfer. *Reprod Biomed Online.* 2014; 28: 310–20.

Chapter 2

The Patient Evaluation of the Future: Genetics, New Diagnostics, and Prediction Modeling

Maurizio Poli, Monica Clemente, Carmen Rubio, Antonio Capalbo, and Carlos Simon

Assessment of the Genetic Risk of a Couple Aiming to Conceive

Genetic risk is defined as the probability of a person (or couple) conceiving a pregnancy with genetic mutations or chromosomal abnormalities that would lead to a severe pathological condition. Genetic mutations are concealed in the genome of almost every person. Most of these mutations are harmless in single copy, but if present in homozygosis, they can lead to severe clinical outcomes. Often, couples carrying unidentified genetic mutations become aware of their dangerous mutations only after conception of an affected child. Around 1300 known recessive genetic conditions have been cataloged to date, affecting over 3 children in every 1000 and accounting for 20% of infant mortality and approximately 10% of pediatric hospitalizations in developed countries[1]. The 20 most common recessive genetic conditions are present in 1–2% of couples of reproductive age, who are thus exposed to a high risk of having a child affected by an inheritable genetic condition.

Total genetic risk of an individual encompasses inheritable conditions, such as mutations or certain chromosomal abnormalities (e.g., Robertsonian translocations), and genetic conditions, whose incidence is not hereditary but age-related (e.g., oocyte chromosomal aneuploidy).

The assessment of genetic risk in prospective parents (partners or patient and donor) through expanded carrier screening (ECS) tests would inform them of the likelihood of transmitting a genetic condition to their offspring. With this knowledge, alternative reproductive/preconception strategies (e.g., IVF+PGT) could be employed to avoid the passing on of a serious genetic condition. Additionally, for conditions where therapeutic interventions are possible, knowledge of carrier status may also allow for preventive and/or timely treatment/intervention, thus reducing morbidity and mortality in affected children.

Single-gene disorders include single-base mutations and triplet expansion genetic abnormalities associated with a pathogenic phenotype. Single-base mutations are commonly referred to as Mendelian traits as their inheritance pattern is completely controlled by one genetic locus, which follows recessive or dominant inheritance (whether autosomal or X-linked). In case of recessivity, the pathology is manifest when both copies of the gene carry the mutation, while in the case of dominance, a single mutated copy is sufficient to generate a pathological condition. An individual is usually aware of carrying a dominant mutation (except for de novo cases or low penetrance conditions) because it is likely to have been previously diagnosed in a family member. However, some dominant mutations (e.g., repeat expansion in dynamic disorders) are not manifest until later in life and direct inheritance may be unclear at the time of conception. These conditions are characterized by expansion and anticipation effect, which entail an increased length of the genetic expansion from one generation to the next, resulting in an earlier onset of the pathology. Similar to trinucleotide repeat disorders, other dominant mutations are not fully penetrant and the link between the presence of the mutation and their actual risk of pathological phenotype might be unpredictable (e.g., neurofibromatosis, NF1). Due to its clear manifestation across family members, mutations characterized by dominant inheritance will be investigated through family history evaluation by a genetic counselor. On the other hand, due to their uncertain pattern of manifestation, late onset and variable penetrance inheritance conditions are not within the scope of reproductive preconception screening and should also be investigated separately with the support of a professional geneticist. The possibility of performing ECS tests on prospective parents (or patient and donor), investigating for the presence of autosomal and X-linked recessive (AR, XLR) mutations clearly linked to pathological conditions, would clarify their genetic risk, enabling an informed choice on the reproductive strategy to undertake.

Certain inheritable conditions are not determined by the presence of a single mutation in a gene but by a combination of genetic and environmental factors that interact in ways not yet fully understood (e.g., type 2 diabetes, Alzheimer's disease, and cancer). The genetic risk associated with a multifactorial condition cannot be precisely estimated as it depends on factors that are not coded in the DNA. However, the presence of certain mutations has been found to be highly associated with an increased risk of developing specific types of cancers (e.g., BRCA 1 and 2 for breast and ovarian cancer). Other genetic mutations involved in multifactorial conditions have been found to give a lower degree of predisposition to the pathology (e.g., BARD1 and BRIP1 for breast and ovarian cancer). Large studies evaluating genome-wide associations (GWAs) are being conducted to improve our understanding of the genetic basis of pathologies and precisely assess the relationship between genomic variants sets and the onset of several pathologies. Regression analysis of these data allows the calculation of polygenic risk scores, which serve as best approximation between the presence of defined multigene variants and the likelihood of developing a specific pathology. Currently, carrier screening testing for multifactorial conditions may not have definitive conclusions regarding the actual risk of onset of a polygenic condition in the offspring, but it may inform on specific predispositions allowing for preventive diagnosis and care. This information is currently given during genetic counseling and family history evaluation consultation sessions.

Most chromosomal abnormalities are incompatible with life, but a small minority of them lead to normal development and lifespan (e.g., balanced Robertsonian translocations), while others, although life-compatible, have appreciable effects on the individual's phenotype (e.g., sexual chromosomes imbalances). Because of their compatibility with life, some aneuploidies may be present in the karyotype of individuals in reproductive age and therefore be transmitted to their offspring. The presence of a balanced or unbalanced translocation in the oocyte or spermatozoon that will form the embryo will determine embryo and fetus' karyotype (normal or abnormal) for that chromosome. The ability to evaluate the presence of structural rearrangements in individuals looking to conceive a baby would determine whether they require ART (and screening of the specific condition in embryos generated through IVF) or if they are not at risk for that determined condition. In this case, the use of ARTs will drastically reduce the chance of miscarriage, fetal death, abnormal conception, and birth defects.

Age-related chromosomal conditions are not inheritable. They are caused by defects in the chromosomal set of germinal cells due to various reasons. The most common one is the accumulation of errors in the meiotic machinery, which results in a significantly inefficient process of germinal cell maturation during meiosis. This defective process is significantly more common in females than males due to the lengthy oocyte maturation progression[2]. According to standard scientific evidence, the number of female germinal cells is determined at birth and from this point in time they suspend their maturational process at an early stage of the first meiosis (dictyotene), which resumes during ovulation. There is solid evidence that the incidence of aneuploidy in embryos generated by women of advanced maternal age is significantly higher than in younger patients. This suggests that the longer the oocytes remain in this suspended maturational state, the higher the chance that the meiotic machinery accumulates defects and is unable to complete the process without resulting in the formation of chromosomal abnormalities. This defective process impacts the ability of females of advanced maternal age to naturally conceive a healthy baby. Since the occurrence of these chromosomal defects is not hereditary, ECS programs cannot precisely identify the risk of an individual generating chromosomally abnormal gametes or embryos. The only effective strategies to assess the presence of nonhereditary chromosomal abnormalities in embryos and fetuses remain preimplantation and prenatal genetic testing. Nonetheless, considerable variability in embryo aneuploidy rates has been reported across women of similar age undergoing preimplantation genetic testing for aneuploidy (PGT-A) cycles. It is therefore possible that part of the genetic determinants of aneuploidy risk may be unraveled in future studies, thus allowing specific risk assessment prior to conception.

Carrier screening platforms have been employed clinically for a few years using different technologies. However, common shortcomings have been the limited knowledge on infrequent genetic diseases and costs associated with multigene testing. A recent study by Haque and colleagues showed that incidence of severe genetic disorders in fetuses is greatly dependent on the parents' ethnic background, with estimated risks ranging between 1:1000 (Hispanic) and 1:250 (Ashkenazi Jewish)[3]. The same study also demonstrated that current ECS panels show significant differences in diagnostic efficacy depending on the ethnical background of the population tested due to a skewed representation of ethnicity-specific mutations[3]. Although possible from a technical point of view, deep multigene assessment has been focused only on the most common pathological conditions due to the high analytical costs associated with parallel multigene analysis. However, this approach left certain ethnicity-specific conditions unscreened, resulting in lower test reliability for certain ethnic groups. Next generation sequencing (NGS) offers the possibility of expanding the breadth of preconception carrier screening capabilities to include a larger number of tested conditions and an increased number of variants investigated, resulting in a more comprehensive diagnostic tool compared to early ethnic-specific carrier screening platforms[4]. Nonetheless, significant differences in the number of conditions tested and their characteristics (e.g., inheritance pathway, severity, penetration, age of onset) and the degree of variant screening efficacy are present in currently available ECS strategies.

As a result, to guarantee an effective preventive strategy for Mendelian disorders at the pre-reproductive stage, careful analysis of the appropriate conditions to be included in the ECS panel should be expertly conducted and diagnostic benchmarks established [5]. In a well-designed ECS gene panel primarily targeting early-onset severe diseases, analytical validity of the tests should be properly investigated to ensure the information generated is reliable in detecting the presence or absence of specific genetic variants. Additionally, clinical validity of variants included in the test should be determined so that presence, absence, or predisposition to the related pathology is clearly established[6].

Therefore, by targeting several areas in the genome, NGS extends coverage of the screening test, drastically reducing residual risk. In this case, testing coverage is defined as the percentage of genetic risk detectable for AR and XLR conditions with an ECS platform. Inversely, residual risk in ECS is defined as the remaining inherent risk after removing the diagnostic information provided by the test.

Although NGS significantly increases the amount of information retrieved to about hundreds or thousands of genes, there are several limitations associated with this approach. For example, NGS may produce false-positive and false-negative findings. Additionally, by producing a detailed map of the whole coding genome when ECS is performed by exome sequencing (ES), much of the data generated may not be presently or unequivocally linked to specific phenotypes or pathological conditions. Moreover, clinical significance of certain complex variants may be uncertain and their association to a pathological phenotype difficult to evaluate, thus impacting on overall clinical validity of the test. For this reason, the characteristics of conditions tested and the scope of the test itself should be carefully considered and expertly reasoned to establish a rational benchmark for providers and patients. With current technology, effective ECS panels can be designed to (1) use systematic principles to include conditions with high prevalence/severity, (2) report pathogenic variants only, and (3) perform with high accuracy[6]. Additionally, growing use of exome/genome sequencing will reveal carrier frequencies for almost every disorder in the tested population, thus improving screening precision and meaningful residual risks calculation.

As discussed above, every person carries a number of mutations that could have drastic effects on the health of their offspring. The implementation of routine ECS is crucial for obtaining a reliable view on each individual genetic risk, allowing patients to make truly informed decisions about their reproductive life. Indeed, serious genetic conditions are recurrently found in the offspring of healthy parents. Studies on the application of ECS testing have revealed that the cumulative risk for healthy individuals to pass on a pathogenic mutation to their children is comparable to the risk for Down's syndrome in the general population[3]. It is therefore possible to anticipate that an increasing number of the population will undergo ECS testing to receive information regarding their genetic risk. However, despite its enormous potential in improving reproductive and postnatal health, ECS platforms still suffer from both technical and diagnostic limitations, which will need exhaustive explanation to prospective patients prior to consenting for testing. In this regard, patients should receive detailed explanation regarding the benefits, risks, and limitations of ECS testing, so that they can make an informed decision on whether to submit to the test. Patients should also be able to decide the level of information they require and whether to include potential late onset conditions (e.g., cancer), low-degree of predisposition to certain pathologies[4].

Additionally, concerns regarding the release of personal genetic information retrieved using ECS to governments or insurers should be leveled by ensuring through legislation (e.g., the Genetic Information Nondiscrimination Act in the United States) that genetic information can be used only in a medical context, whether to prevent, treat, or avoid a pathological condition, but never to discriminate against individuals from a financial or legal standpoint.

As technology develops, it will be possible to assemble ECS panels that test for the most serious and common genetic conditions, leaving minimal residual risk. With parallel reduction in cost per analysis, ECS testing should become more affordable for patients favoring an extensive implementation in clinical routine. Additionally, ongoing GWA studies will likely improve overall clinical utility of ECS testing further progressing prediction, prevention, and treatment of an increasing number of genetic conditions. Similar to other forms of preventive screening, the ECS panel is likely to become a crucial tool for pathological investigation and treatment design. With the evolution of pharmacogenomics, ECS data will provide key information for enabling true personalized medicine, including administration of most effective drugs and dosages, predicting drug response or toxicity, and avoiding the application of ineffective or suboptimal treatment regimens. Notably, a single whole exome sequencing analysis would enable personalized medical intervention for the whole life by allowing retrospective evaluation of the sequencing data against most up-to-date genomic findings.

Assessing Endometrial Receptivity Using Prediction Models

The endometrial factor plays a key role in the reproductive process as a receptive endometrium is necessary for embryo implantation. The limited period in which the embryo can attach to the maternal endometrium is known as the window of implantation (WOI). Identifying an individual's WOI allows for the synchronization of endometrial receptivity with an embryo ready to implant in a personalized embryo transfer (pET). This strategy improves outcomes of assisted reproduction for women with recurrent implantation failure (RIF)[7].

Commonly, histological criteria have been employed to date the endometrium. However, morphological criteria have major limitations in predicting endometrial receptivity, as demonstrated in randomized studies[8]. Endometrial receptivity has also been unsuccessfully investigated using several single markers[9].

Over the last decade, transcriptomics has emerged as a powerful tool in diagnosing disease and determining prognosis. The reproductive field is not an exception and the transcriptomics of the human endometrium has been widely investigated[10]. The main interest has focused on the identification of the specific transcriptomic signature that can identify a receptive endometrial function and improve the effectiveness of reproductive treatments.

Endometrial receptivity analysis (ERA) was the first transcriptomic test introducing the concept of pET by timing ET according to each patient's personalized WOI (pWOI) [7,11]. Although most women reach receptivity after five full days of progesterone administration, some of them are affected by WOI displacement. Application of ERA revealed that 25% of patients experiencing RIF had a displaced WOI, with a faster or slower response to progesterone, leading to asynchrony between embryo and endometrium. Therefore, it is very important to identify a specific WOI for each patient to synchronize the transfer of a viable blastocyst with a receptive endometrium. ERA testing has been clinically applied since 2010, and different groups around the world have reported its clinical results[12,13].

ERA was initially developed as a microarray-based clinical test measuring the transcriptomic signature of 238 genes to assess endometrium receptive status[11]. This customized microarray was coupled with a computational predictor able to identify the specific transcriptomic profile for each endometrial stage, namely proliferative (PRO), pre-receptive (PRE), receptive (R), and post-receptive (POST).

Recently, an increasing number of researchers are choosing NGS over microarray for transcriptomics investigations. The use of a sequencing technology that delivers fast, cost accessible, and accurate transcriptomic information has motivated the chapter authors' team to move from microarray-based ERA to NGS-based ERA 2.0.

ERA 2.0 is a predictor tool based on a machine-learning classification model[14]. Classification models are supervised learning methods for predicting the value of a categorical target attribute. Models are developed using a set of past observations whose target class is known and a set of explanatory variables. A prediction (class probability) is obtained by applying the model to new samples.

Specifically, the explanatory variables are the ERA genes counts obtained by sequencing files and the categorical attribute to predict is the different endometrial receptivity profiles. In summary, our objective was to identify the different endometrial stages using the transcriptomic profile determined by the original ERA genes. The identified profile gives indications on how to adjust progesterone administration to reach optimal endometrial receptivity: pre-receptive requiring 2 extra days (PREd2), pre-receptive requiring 1 extra day (PREd1), early receptive requiring 12 extra hours (ER), R, late receptive requiring 12 hours less (LR), POST requiring 1 day less, or PRO, which would imply absence of progesterone in the endometrium or a lack in response to it.

In a classification task, it is very important to select well-defined and curated samples to train the predictor model. This was warranted by the chapter authors' expertise acquired through the analysis of over 20 000 endometrial samples worldwide.

The data set for NGS predictor development comprised 411 endometrial biopsies in which ERA was previously diagnosed by microarray technology. This data covered all the different profiles: PREd2, PREd1, ER, R, LR, POST, and PRO. The receptive group included samples with successful pregnancy after pET, while the nonreceptive group comprised samples with a second ERA biopsy reaching receptivity after WOI correction based on first ERA recommendation. This dataset comprised women with a mean age of 37.5 ± 5 years old (mean +/- standard deviation), with BMI mean of 23.3 ± 3.6 Kg/m^2. Most of the samples were taken in hormone replacement therapy (HRT) cycles (82%), while the remaining were taken in natural cycles.

These data were randomly split into training set (70% of data set) and test set (30% of data set). The training set was used for building the classification model (n=290 samples), and the test set (n=121) was used to provide an unbiased performance evaluation.

During algorithm development, several models were studied to find those most appropriate for our data. Four of the most popular machine-learning algorithm methods for classification problems were compared: support vector machine, k-nearest neighbor, random forest (RF), and classification tree[15]. Optimal tuning parameters for each model were selected based on a resampling technique (a repeated k-fold cross-validation).

The performance of each model was computed over the test set in terms of global accuracy, sensitivity, and specificity. After comparing all models, the RF obtained the best results with an accuracy of 0.88 (95% CI 0.80–0.92). As we had more than two classes, the performance was calculated from "one-versus-all"; the mean sensitivity was 0.90 and mean specificity was 0.97.

The predictor identified when the endometrium reached receptivity during the cycle. So, if a first ERA was done at the expected day of WOI (progesterone (P) + 5, luteinizing hormone (LH) + 7, or human chorionic gonadotropin (hCG) + 7) with a nonreceptive result, a second endometrial biopsy was recommended on the day predicted by ERA 2.0.

An analysis was performed using paired-biopsies verification compound by 1 432 endometrial samples (n=716 paired samples). The first biopsy of these paired biopsies was predicted to need one more day of progesterone administration (diagnosed as PREd1). A successful match was considered when the patient followed the ERA recommendation and the result of the second biopsy was R, or if the patient did not follow the ERA recommendation and the result was nonreceptive (NR) (as expected).

The paired biopsy verification analysis was evaluated in terms of percentage of prediction success after a second biopsy. Out of the 716 PREd1 paired samples, the success proportion was 0.89 (95% CI 0.86–0.91).

Figure 2.1 shows the workflow followed to identify the endometrial receptivity by the ERA 2.0 test.

Clinical follow-up after pET based on ERA NGS predictor in 261 RIF patients (age: 37.3±5.1) from 5 clinics was performed[14]. Data were reported as pregnancy rate (PR) (percentage of patients with βhCG positive over the total of patients with pET), implantation rate (IR) (percentage of gestational sacs observed by vaginal ultrasound at fifth week post-transfer over the number of transferred embryos), and ongoing pregnancy rate (OPR) (percentage of ongoing pregnancies at twelfth week over total of patients with pET). These results showed 70.9% PR, 55.7% IR, and 59.4% OPR.

In summary, embryo implantation is a complex process that involves different players, among which endometrial receptivity is one. Although most women reach endometrial receptivity on the same days after ovulation or during secretory phase in an HRT treatment, some of them show a displaced WOI. Transcriptomic analysis has enabled the study of how gene expression changes at different endometrial stages and has been instrumental in the understanding of the WOI.

The identification of the pWOI in RIF patients has provided a recommendation for pET leading to an improvement in pregnancy and implantation rates.

New technological achievements in the area of transcriptomics, combined with our ERA know-how after more than 20 000 patients analyzed, have motivated the

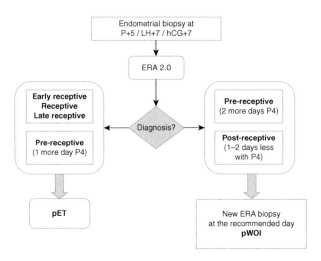

Figure 2.1 Workflow employed for the identification of receptivity in an endometrial sample

development of new predictor ERA 2.0. The ERA 2.0 combines NGS technology (based on the original gene panel) and a predictor trained according to our ERA expertise. The knowledge acquired during these years has helped to refine ERA diagnostic profiles by using well-defined samples (with known clinical outcome/validated prediction). The paired biopsy verification showed that, in the case of samples first diagnosed as PREd1, the prediction allows an accurate pET recommendation. These results could help doctors concerning the convenience of performing a second biopsy in the case of a first non-receptive result. Interestingly, 90% of samples received at our facilities were receptive (R, ER, LR) or PREd1.

The change to NGS and the development of a new ERA predictor has led to an improvement in diagnostic accuracy, reaching better clinical outcomes compared to other publications with ERA microarray-based predictor. A PR in a range of 50–51.7% and IR of 33.9–38.5% was reported in RIF patients when pET was performed according to the pWOI of the patient[7], versus the current published outcome of 70.9% PR and 55.7% IR obtained with ERA 2.0.

In conclusion, our results demonstrate that ERA NGS combined with machine-learning methods based on our wide ERA know-how enhances pWOI detection accuracy and clinical effectiveness, significantly improving reproductive outcomes when pET is performed.

Noninvasive Preimplantation Aneuploidy Testing: Embryonic Cell Free DNA in the Spent Blastocyst Medium

The most common genetic abnormality identified in human embryos is aneuploidy. This abnormality is particularly common among embryos produced by IVF – more than half are aneuploid[16]. Hence, analyzing chromosomal status of the embryo using PGT-A enables embryo selection that can result in better pregnancy rates in infertile couples requiring ART. PGT-A using comprehensive techniques to test for all 24 chromosomes has improved clinical outcomes. NGS in trophectoderm (TE) biopsies is the technology most widely applied nowadays. This technology is also susceptible to the detection of different grades of mosaicism in TE biopsy and there are now concerns related to the real incidence of mosaicism in preimplantation embryos due to technical and biological limitations in a TE biopsy, since it represents a small percentage of the total number of cells of the blastocyst. Also, the potential harm to the blastocyst during biopsy has prevented some clinicians implementing PGT-A in some IVF programs.

The primary aim of ARTs is to help patients in achieving a pregnancy that ends in a healthy baby at home. For that purpose, identifying the embryos with the highest potential to implant and establish ongoing pregnancy is crucial. It is known that euploid embryos are the ones with the highest implantation potential and OPRs. Aneuploid embryos can reach the blastocyst stage and, depending on the type of aneuploidy, some of them will not implant, others will implant into the uterus but will end in a miscarriage, and others, few of them, can result in an affected newborn. The identification of aneuploidies is especially important in embryos from patients with higher aneuploidy risk such as those with advanced maternal age, RIF, recurrent miscarriage or SMF[17]. Besides, these aneuploid blastocysts could have a very good morphology[18]. Therefore, determining the chromosome complement of the blastocyst is the key limiting factor to know whether an embryo will develop into a chromosomally normal newborn.

In PGT-A, the full chromosome content of a single or few cells is analyzed with high sensitivity and specificity. However, the input material is obtained by an invasive method: a biopsy. Therefore, PGT-A involves a high investment for the IVF laboratory as, to carry out the biopsy, specialized equipment like a laser is required and, in addition, this procedure must be conducted by trained embryologists also to avoid operator-dependent bias in the results. Recently, there have been different attempts to overcome biopsy to diagnose the chromosomal content of the embryos. Some groups started with the analysis of blastocoel fluid obtained by aspiration with a thin micropipette as a less invasive approach than TE biopsy. This technique, known as blastocentesis, needs to be conducted in expanded blastocysts, taking especial care in avoiding aspiration of any cellular material that would contaminate the sample. The volume of DNA retrieved is very low (less than 1 µl) and its quantity and integrity limit further analysis. This can be seen in the different publications on the topic where, despite having amplification rates higher than 60% in all cases, the concordance rates for aneuploidy were very variable among them: from 48%[19] to 97.1%[20].

Later on, some groups proposed a "true" noninvasive approach consisting in the study of the spent culture media to analyze the embryonic cell-free DNA (cfDNA) released by the embryo during the latest stages of preimplantation development. After the first publications, several studies have compared the results of PGT-A in TE biopsies with the results of the spent culture media to establish the concordance rates among both approaches. All studies were able to obtain high amplification rates for the cfDNA, ranging from 80 to 100%. However, there were highly variable concordance rates among them: 3.5% on a proof-of-concept study[21], 85.7%[22], 72.2% [23], 30.4%[24], and 65%[25]. The discrepancies in the reported results could be related to the different methodologies applied regarding embryo culture (culture drop volume and time in culture) blastocyst manipulation (assisted hatching, vitrification), and DNA analysis (amplification and detection methods), as well as to the different criteria used to define the concordance rates. How the embryo is handled during the whole process is extremely important because it can determine not only the quantity and quality of the DNA present in the spent culture medium but also the presence of residual cumulus cells not completely removed from the oocyte, which could lead to contamination with maternal DNA, resulting in false negatives.

Furthermore, in another study the results of the combination of blastocoel fluid and spent culture medium were compared with TE biopsy and with the whole blastocysts. This study found higher concordance rates between media and whole blastocyst embryo than between the TE and the whole blastocyst, pointing out that blastocoel fluid and spent culture medium could be more representative of the "true" chromosomal content of the embryos than trophectoderm[26].

In a recent study, the chapter authors compared the informativity and concordance rates of TE biopsies with the analysis of the cfDNA in the culture media. In this study, the embryos were not previously subjected to assisted hatching, blastocentesis, or any vitrification or biopsy procedure, with intact zona pellucida. Our goal was to validate a "true" noninvasive PGT-A method to identify the chromosomal status of the embryos by analyzing the embryonic cfDNA without the need of a biopsy. In a pilot study, encouraging results were produced, with high informativity rates, when the blastocyst media were collected after 48 hours in culture and with 84.0% concordance rate with the TE biopsy[27].

A noninvasive approach to study the chromosomal status of embryos could have several important advantages when compared to current invasive PGT-A with TE biopsy. First, avoiding invasiveness with potential embryo harm, while extending the feasibility of PGT-A in a larger number of clinics and increasing its accessibility from a wider population of patients by minimizing laboratory and personnel expenses. Therefore, this approach would be accessible worldwide. Most importantly, we may improve on the diagnostic uncertainty regarding TE biopsy and mosaicism. TE biopsies are surely representative of meiotic errors. However, for detection of mitotic errors and the understanding of mosaicism, new sources of DNA such as embryonic cfDNA, which is potentially released by the cells of the whole embryo, could provide additional valuable information and help to elucidate the real impact of mosaicism on clinical outcomes. Further clinical studies and more basic research would be needed to fully address the remaining questions related to the origin of the cfDNA, its representativeness of the full embryo chromosome content, and its potential clinical applications to improve IVF outcomes.

Genomics and the Future of Personalized Reproductive Medicine

Genomics approaches are already being employed to determine and quantify the reproductive fitness of patients undergoing IVF treatments. These diagnostic/prognostic tools target both the embryo in terms of chromosomal content and presence of mutations, and the endometrium in terms of transcriptional patterns. Additionally, all individuals trying to conceive (whether naturally or through IVF) can now be assessed for the presence of common recessive mutations that may be inherited by the ensuing baby. In fact, in the presence of pathological mutations, carrier screening can provide crucial knowledge on couples' reproductive risk, allowing for timely considerations of safer reproductive alternatives (e.g., IVF+PGT).

Presently, the combination of these three approaches has the potential to improve IVF treatment outcomes, while eliminating the risk of abnormal conception and reducing the chance of miscarriage.

Nonetheless, certain forms of infertility cannot be identified through anatomical or endocrinological assessment and fall under the "unexplained infertility" definition. These cases are treated with standard protocols even though their root causes can be extremely diverse. Future global application of preconception genome and ES will further improve reproductive diagnostic and prognostic tools. Through large genome-wide association studies genetic variants causing infertility will eventually be identified, thus not only increasing knowledge of molecular pathways of embryo development and implantation but also providing personalized reproductive prognostics and tailored infertility treatment and management for each individual couple or patient.

References

1. Kumar P, Radhakrishnan J, Chowdhary MA, Giampietro PF. Prevalence and Patterns of Presentation of Genetic Disorders in a Pediatric Emergency Department. *Mayo Clin Proc.* 2018; 76(**8**): 777–83.

2. Capalbo A, Hoffmann ER, Cimadomo D, Maria Ubaldi F, Rienzi L. Human Female Meiosis Revised: New Insights into the Mechanisms of Chromosome Segregation and Aneuploidies from Advanced Genomics and Time-Lapse Imaging. *Hum Reprod Update.* 2017; 23(**6**): 706–22.

3. Haque IS, Lazarin GA, Kang HP, Evans EA, Goldberg JD, Wapner RJ. Modeled Fetal Risk of Genetic Diseases Identified by Expanded Carrier Screening. *JAMA.* 2016; 316(**7**): 734.

4. Grody WW, Thompson BH, Gregg AR, Bean LH, Monaghan KG, Schneider A, et al. ACMG Position Statement on Prenatal/Preconception Expanded Carrier Screening. *Genet Med.* 2018; 15(**6**): 482–3.

5. Burke W. Genetic Tests: Clinical Validity and Clinical Utility. *Curr Protoc Hum Genet.* 2014; 81(**9.15**): 1–8.

6. Hogan GJ, Vysotskaia VS, Beauchamp KA, Seisenberger S, Grauman PV, Haas KR, et al. Validation of an Expanded Carrier Screen That Optimizes Sensitivity Via Full-Exon Sequencing and Panel-Wide Copy Number Variant Identification. *Clin Chem.* 2018; 64(**7**): 1063–73.

7. Ruíz-Alonso M, Blesa D, Díaz-Gimeno P, Gómez E, Fernández-Sánchez M, Carranza F, et al. The Endometrial Receptivity Array for Diagnosis and Personalized Embryo Transfer As a Treatment for Patients with Repeated Implantation Failure. *Fertil Steril.* 2013; 100(**3**): 818–24.

8. Coutifaris C, Myers ER, Guzick DS, Diamond MP, Carson SA, Legro RS, et al. Histological Dating of Timed Endometrial Biopsy Tissue Is Not Related to Fertility Status. *Fertil Steril.* 2004; 82(**5**): 1264–72.

9. Aghajanova L, Hamilton AE, Giudice LC. Uterine Receptivity to Human Embryonic Implantation: Histology, Biomarkers, and Transcriptomics. *Semin Cell Dev Biol.* 2018; 19(**2**): 204–11.

10. Díaz-Gimeno P, Ruíz-Alonso M, Blesa D, Simón C. Transcriptomics of the Human Endometrium. *Int J Dev Biol.* 2014; 58 (**2–3–4**): 127–37.

11. Díaz-Gimeno P, Horcajadas JA, Martínez-Conejero JA, Esteban FJ, Alamá P, Pellicer A, et al. A Genomic Diagnostic Tool for Human Endometrial Receptivity Based on the Transcriptomic Signature. *Fertil Steril.* 2011; 95(**1**): 50–60.

12. Hashimoto T, Koizumi M, Doshida M, Toya M, Sagara E, Oka N, et al. Efficacy of the Endometrial Receptivity Array for Repeated Implantation Failure in Japan: A Retrospective, Two-Centers Study. *Reprod Med Biol.* 2017; 16(**3**): 290–6.

13. Tan J, Kan A, Hitkari J, Taylor B, Tallon N, Warraich G, et al. The Role of the Endometrial Receptivity Array (Era) in Patients Who Have Failed Euploid Embryo Transfers. *J Assist Reprod Genet.* 2018; 35(**4**): 683–92.

14. Clemente-Ciscar M, Ruíz-Alonso M, Blesa D, Jimenez-Almazan J, Al E. Endometrial Receptivity Analysis (ERA) Using a Next Generation Sequencing

(NGS) Predictor Improves Reproductive Outcome in Recurrent Implantation Failure. In: *Abstracts of the 34rd Annual Meeting of the European Society of Human Reproduction and Embryology*. 2018.

15. Friedman J, Hastie T, Tibshirani R. The Elements of Statistical Learning. New York: Springer Series in Statistics. 2001.

16. Franasiak JM, Forman EJ, Hong KH, Werner MD, Upham KM, Treff NR, et al. Aneuploidy Across Individual Chromosomes at the Embryonic Level in Trophectoderm Biopsies: Changes with Patient Age and Chromosome Structure. *J Assist Reprod Genet*. 2018; 31(**11**): 1501–9.

17. Rodrigo L, Mateu E, Mercader A, Cobo AC, Peinado V, Milán M, et al. New Tools for Embryo Selection: Comprehensive Chromosome Screening by Array Comparative Genomic Hybridization. *Biomed Res Int*. 2014; 2014: 517125.

18. Alfarawati S, Fragouli E, Colls P, Stevens J, Gutiérrez-Mateo C, Schoolcraft WB, et al. The Relationship Between Blastocyst Morphology, Chromosomal Abnormality, and Embryo Gender. *Fertil Steril*. 2011; 95 (**2**): 520–4.

19. Tobler KJ, Zhao Y, Ross R, Benner AT, Xu X, Du L, et al. Blastocoel Fluid from Differentiated Blastocysts Harbors Embryonic Genomic Material Capable of a Whole-Genome Deoxyribonucleic Acid Amplification and Comprehensive Chromosome Microarray Analysis. *Fertil Steril*. 2015; 104(**2**): 418–25.

20. Gianaroli L, Magli MC, Pomante A, Crivello AM, Cafueri G, Valerio M, et al. Blastocentesis: A Source of DNA for Preimplantation Genetic Testing. Results from a Pilot Study. *Fertil Steril*. 2018; 102 (**6**): 1692–9.e6.

21. Shamonki MI, Jin H, Haimowitz Z, Liu L. Proof of Concept: Preimplantation Genetic Screening Without Embryo Biopsy through Analysis of Cell-Free DNA in Spent Embryo Culture Media. *Fertil Steril*. 2016; 106(**6**): 1312–18.

22. Xu J, Fang R, Chen L, Chen D, Xiao J-P, Yang W, et al. Noninvasive Chromosome Screening of Human Embryos by Genome Sequencing of Embryo Culture Medium for in Vitro Fertilization. *Proc Natl Acad Sci USA*. 2016; 113(**42**): 11907–12.

23. Feichtinger M, Vaccari E, Carli L, Wallner E, Mädel U, Figl K, et al. Non-Invasive Preimplantation Genetic Screening Using Array Comparative Genomic Hybridization on Spent Culture Media: A Proof-of-Concept Pilot Study. *Reprod Biomed Online*. 2017; 34(**6**): 583–9.

24. Vera-Rodriguez M, Rubio C. Assessing the True Incidence of Mosaicism in Preimplantation Embryos. *Fertil Steril*. 2017; 107(**5**): 1107–12.

25. Ho JR, Arrach N, Rhodes-Long K, Ahmady A, Ingles S, Chung K, et al. Pushing the Limits of Detection: Investigation of Cell-Free DNA for Aneuploidy Screening in Embryos. *Fertil Steril*. 2018; 110(**3**): 467–475.e2.

26. Kuznyetsov V, Madjunkova S, Antes R, Abramov R, Motamedi G, Ibarrientos Z, et al. Evaluation of a Novel Non-Invasive Preimplantation Genetic Screening Approach. *PLoS One*. 2018; 13(**5**): e0197262.

27. Rubio C, Rienzi L, Navarro-Sánchez L, Cimadomo D, García-Pascual C, Soscia D, et al. Origin of False Positives and False Negatives in Non-Invasive Preimplantation Genetic Testing for Aneuploidies. In: *ASRM Denver*; *Fertil Steril*. 2018.

Chapter 3

Advances in ART Pharmacology: Drug Delivery Systems and the Pipeline

Colin M Howles

Introduction

Since the very early years (1969–1978) of human IVF, Patrick Steptoe and Robert Edwards were utilizing a range of pharmaceutical agents for ovarian stimulation, ovulation induction, and luteal phase support (e.g., urinary gonadotrophins, chorionic gonadotrophin, clomiphene citrate, progesterone)[1,2]. However, in spite of their efforts with these agents, their breakthrough pregnancy following ovarian stimulation was sadly an ectopic[3]. After this setback, the pioneering team decided to revert to natural cycle IVF, and the first IVF birth, Louise Brown, marked the end of the beginning of human IVF[4]. However, soon after there was broad recognition from the first IVF groups around the globe that "ovarian stimulation promised more oocytes and therefore more pregnancies, and (would) allow a better scheduling of oocyte collection[5]."

While there has been, over the years, a forward and backwards debate in the literature and international conferences on the issue of mild stimulation/natural cycle regimens versus conventional controlled ovarian stimulation protocols[6,7], data from both country registries and multicenter initiatives now demonstrate that the number of oocytes recovered is directly correlated with the cumulative live birth rate when vitrified embryos are also considered[8,9]. Today, we are fortunate to have a large armament of pharmaceutical agents to utilize in ART protocols. However, drug choice, dosing regimens, and modes of administration are highly variable and dependent on patient, clinical, and geographical variables. Injectable gonadotrophins have evolved from crude, and then more refined, urinary preparations[10], to highly purified recombinant human (r-h) gonadotrophins; the latter being available in pen devices, which allow a wide range of doses to be utilized (more background on the evolution can be found in Ludwig et al. and Lunenfeld[11,12]).

Drug development is a highly complex and regulated process, which is both costly and has a high failure rate. It has been stated that to get one drug approval an average of 8.5 compounds need to be put through clinical development[13]. Additionally, in reproductive medicine the ART treatment process is in itself highly complex and subject to multiple variables emanating from the patient, clinical, and laboratory procedures. Often the primary drug-related (pharmacodynamic) endpoint can be remote from the desired treatment endpoint. For example, the most important pharmaceutical drug utilized in an ART treatment is follicle-stimulating hormone (FSH), which is responsible for the growth and development of the ovarian follicle from which a mature oocyte will be aspirated. However, the desired treatment outcome is a healthy baby, which is dependent primarily on upstream (patient) as well as downstream laboratory and clinical procedures[14]. Thus, there is an important disconnect between FSH drug action and ART treatment outcome, which raises additional challenges for the drug developers, especially when dealing with different regulatory authorities (e.g., the United States FDA routinely demand clinical pregnancy as a primary endpoint for gonadotrophins).

The ART therapeutic area, while growing at around 10% in treatment cycles per year [15], is still, in medical terms, relatively small. It is estimated that the total number of ART treatment cycles worldwide is around two million[16]. This compares, for example, with the therapeutic area of diabetes where in the United States alone, 9.4% of the population have diabetes and 1.5 million are diagnosed each year, with need of insulin therapy.

Additionally, as far as ovarian stimulation is concerned, the period of treatment is relatively short (i.e., for FSH with/without LH median 11 days)[17].

The following sections will give a brief overview of the drug development process: challenges and potential opportunities specific to ART, modes of delivery for gonadotrophins, gonadotropin-releasing hormone (GnRH) analogs, and luteal phase supporting drugs, with some insights on in-development or recently launched therapeutics.

Drug Development Can Be a Long and Risky Business

It has been estimated that developing a new prescription medicine that enters the clinic costs the pharmaceutical industry around $2.6 billion USD[13,18]. DiMasi and colleagues[18] used information provided by 10 pharmaceutical companies on 106 randomly selected drugs that were first tested in human subjects anywhere in the world from 1995 to 2007. This represents a 145% increase from the previous study carried out 10 years previously. Additionally, although the average time taken to bring a drug through clinical trials has actually decreased, the rate of success has gone down by almost one-half, to just 12%. This study has naturally had its critics and some commentators refer to a previous study carried out by the Office of Health Economics[19], which provided an estimate of $1.5 billion USD (at 2011 prices).

However, all authors agree that costs have dramatically increased requiring clinical trials of increasing complexity, which are a crucial part of the drug development process. Such trials (ranging from phase I, II, III to postapproval IV) have to be conducted to demonstrate drug safety and efficacy so that approval for clinical use can be obtained

Table 3.1 Examples of drug development time in reproductive medicine therapy area

Molecule	Patent issued	First scientific publication	Clinical development time[1] (phase I–III)	First regulatory registration
FSH (recombinant)	1988	1989	1992–1995 (4 years)	1996 (Europe)
FSH (recombinant biosimilar)	No patent	2015	2009–2013 (5 years)	2014 (Europe)
FSH (recombinant long-acting fusion carboxyl terminal peptide (CTP))	1989	1992	2001–2008 (8 years)	2010 (Europe)
GnRH analog (antagonist)	1980	1986	1991–1997 (7 years)	1999 (Europe)
GnRH antagonist (orally active small molecule)	1987	1989	2010–2017 (8 years)	2018 (United States)

[1] Calculated from time of publications

from regulatory bodies. The cost of carrying out clinical trials varies according to therapeutic area, size of the pharmaceutical company, and whether the test molecule is a chemical compound or a biologic (e.g., FSH) and also between different development phases. In the United States, the highest cost of clinical trials is in the respiratory system therapeutic area ($115 million USD), while for the endocrine area, the clinical trial costs are estimated to be around $59.1 million USD including the regulatory review phase. Table 3.1 gives some examples of the research and development time for some of the FSH and GnRH antagonist drugs used in the reproductive medicine field. The fastest was for a recombinant form of natural human follicle stimulating hormone (hFSH) (from patent to registration: 9 years) compared with 30 years for orally active GnRH antagonist. The reasons for these widely differing time frames are many and some will be discussed in this chapter.

Another important element to consider that is particularly relevant to the ART therapeutic area is the rise in importance of "biotech" companies and how they are today feeding "big pharma" with innovative candidate products to replenish their drug pipelines. In the last months of 2018/2019, three big pharmaceutical companies splashed out almost $100 billion USD in deals, which brought biotechs little-known outside Silicon Valley or Cambridge, Massachusetts, under their wings (*Financial Times*, January 11, 2019). The characteristics of these two players are summarized in Table 3.2.

Table 3.2 Main characteristics of traditional pharmaceutical and biotech companies

Characteristic	Pharmaceutical	Biotech
Size	Large organization	Small, often spun out of academic research
Presence	Wide global footprint	Country/regional presence
Core competences	Research, develop, manufacture, and market drugs	"pure research engine"
Technologies primarily used	Empirical screening techniques	Use genetic engineering
Value	Cash rich – high overheads	Cash poor – mixture of private and public funding: low overheads

Biologic drugs, examples of which in ART are the recombinant (a core strength of biotech companies) and urinary gonadotrophins, are produced using a biological source. Increasingly, these complex glycoproteins are derived using genetically engineered cells [10]. The glycoproteins naturally exist in a range of forms (isoforms) due to subtle differences in the carbohydrate moieties, which are attached to the protein backbone. In spite of the inherent variability in the isoform profile between different marketed recombinant and urinary gonadotrophin FSH preparations, they all essentially have the same therapeutic features, reflected in similar daily dosing regimens and length of treatment.

An important milestone in gonadotrophin development was the first birth following stimulation of follicular growth in a hypopituitary hypogonadal woman (WHO group I) with recombinant human FSH (r-hFSH) as well as recombinant human luteinizing hormone (r-hLH) and then recombinant human chorionic gonadotropin (r-hCG) to induce final follicular maturation and ovulation[20], signaling that the era of all recombinant gonadotrophins had truly commenced.

Over a 25-year period, there have been numerous attempts to demonstrate the benefit of "LH activity" in ART patients. However, these have not translated into regulatory approval for the clinical use of a r-hLH/r-hFSH combination product. While there seems to be some physiological rationale as to the potential benefit of LH in low responders/ women of advanced maternal age, the largest randomized controlled trials (RCTs) to date demonstrated no benefit of LH supplementation in terms of oocytes or pregnancy outcomes[21].

Recently, r-hFSH preparations have become available in the European Union (EU) – the so-called "biosimilars" – which bear essentially the same active pharmaceutical ingredient (API) to be used at the same dose, via the same route for the same indications as the reference medicinal product, in this case follitropin alfa (Gonal-f, Merck KGaA, Darmstadt), which was first registered in 1996[22].

In 2005, the European Medicines Agency put forward a stringent regulatory framework for biosimilars development, which became the foundation for other regulatory bodies around the world including the United States FDA who initiated such a pathway in 2015[23]. The biosimilars have biologic activity comparable to their corresponding reference drugs and are often more cost-effective. To stimulate innovation and new market entrants, the regulatory pathway allows for the biosimilar to extrapolate and "piggyback" on the branded biological to get approval for all the original drug's indications. Even so, it can still take somewhere between 5 and 9 years to develop a biosimilar at a cost of $100–250 million USD[24]. This compares with a development time of about 2 years and a cost of $1–2 million USD for a small-molecule generic. Bringing a biosimilar to the market is not for the fainthearted!

The Use and Delivery of FSH Biologics in Reproductive Medicine

Until the general availability of recombinant gonadotrophins, all urinary preparations were available in a lyophilized form, either in a glass ampoule (which needed to be snapped open by the patient or nurse) or in a vial with a rubber stopper to allow a needle to be pushed through for the next step. Additionally, the very first products (first-generation urinaries) had low specific activity and required to be injected intramuscularly until the availability of highly purified urinary FSH[25]. These formulations also required reconstitution steps, and the use of different syringes/needles than those for injection, which undoubtedly played a role in increasing the potential for injection errors, which could affect pregnancy outcome[26,27,28].

A major step forward, though, as far as patient convenience, ease of use, and facilitating the teaching process of drug administration for the health-care professional, was the availability of recombinant gonadotrophins as a liquid formulation and finally in prefilled pen devices[29,30,31].

In a variety of country and multinational studies[32,33], it was documented that over half the patients interviewed reported ovarian stimulation had an impact on their day-to-day lifestyle, in particular regarding whether the correct daily dose had been administered correctly. Thus, the availability of a delivery device which provides patients with attributes that assist in minimizing the impact on their daily life and simplifies the ease of teaching for health-care professionals (in particular nurses) is the desired goal. A recent multicenter study, which was designed to assess such product specific features of a range of self-administered FSH injection devices used in ART, clearly demonstrated important differences between injection devices, which were shared across users in a number of European countries[31]. Overall, for both patients and nurses, the ideal FSH injection device would be a highly accurate, multiuse pen injector, with a dial-back function which is easy to use and/or teach. These attributes are present with one of the recently available biosimilar FSH devices (Ovaleap, Theramex, UK).

It has been well documented that the most frequent cause for patients to drop out from IVF treatment is the physical or psychological burden of the treatment process [34]. Daily injections can be far more distressing for a patient than health-care professionals realize[35]. Another approach was taken by one drug manufacturer (Organon, now Merck, Sharp, and Dohme [MSD]) to address these patients' concerns; namely to reduce the burden (number) of injections required by utilizing a recombinant fusion molecule (corifollitropin alfa). The initial design for this molecule was conceptualized in the early 1990s by Irving Biome's research group in St. Louis, Missouri, United States

[36]. Here, human FSH is coupled to the CTP of hCG, which naturally extends FSH's half-life in human serum (to around 70 hours compared with that of follitropin alfa or beta of around 36–40 hours). Because of the extended absorption and longer half-life of corifollitropin alfa, the frequency of FSH administration may be reduced, resulting in more injection-free days for patients undergoing controlled ovarian stimulation (COS).

The first live birth after ovarian stimulation using r-hFSH-CTP was reported by Beckers and colleagues[37] and the molecule was registered in the EU for use in ART in 2010. Two dose forms are available: 100 µg for women with body weight ≤60 kg and 150 µg FSH-CTP for women with body weight >60 kg.

Following its introduction in the EU (2010), corifollitropin alfa did not really live up to initial expectations. In September 2013, Merck & Co (MSD outside of United States) announced that a new drug application was accepted for review by the United States FDA. Just 10 months later in July 2014, Merck & Co announced the receipt of a complete response letter from the United States FDA. In the Merck & Co annual report[38], it was stated that the company had "made a decision to discontinue development of corifollitropin alfa injection in the United States for business reasons."

The reasons for the drug's lackluster performance are probably numerous; the first being that longer-acting drugs are more suited for chronic disease conditions. The impact of reducing the number of injections during a COS cycle was, I believe, limited due to the fact that other injections (daily GnRH antagonist injections) still had to be administered, so there were in effect only 3–4 injection-free days compared to standard daily treatment. Additionally, as an injection of corifollitropin alfa was developed to be active for just seven days, if the appropriate follicular response had not been achieved by that time, daily FSH injections would then need to be administered, thus a patient may have to learn two injection techniques for FSH in one treatment cycle. The use of this novel drug also led to different follicular growth dynamics, which may not have fitted some clinical units' procedures.

Finally, it must also be remembered that, due to the long elimination half-life after subcutaneous injection of 36–40 hours[39] of standard r-hFSH, it is feasible to reduce injection frequency to every three days if desired[40]. Alternate-day FSH regimens have been previously described both for ovulation induction and ART[41], but never really caught on, probably due to concerns around injection compliance.

MSD is now focusing development efforts in applying corifollitropin alfa in a chronic condition: the treatment of male hypogonadism[42]. In this condition, it is first necessary to restore testosterone levels back into the normal range with hCG alone for 3–6 months [43], before moving to combination therapy with 2–3 times weekly FSH injections for up to 18 months if spermatogenesis is the desired outcome.

A major learning from this is that, while the drug treatment burden can be an important barrier, the available pen device systems for daily administration probably provide sufficient confidence to the vast majority of patients when faced with a relatively short FSH treatment duration of around 11 days.

Another recombinant human FSH (follitropin delta; Rekovelle Ferring Pharmaceuticals) with different pharmacokinetic properties compared to existing FSH products, was granted marketing authorization by the European Commission in December 2016. In view of its longer elimination half-life (30 hours versus 24 hours for follitropin alfa[44]), due to follitropin delta's higher overall sialic acid content, the product is dosed based on AMH and weight (kg) of the IVF patient[45]. This product is again available in a multidose pen device for daily injections of the same individualized dose based on the measurement of AMH from only one validated assay system and weight. While follitropin delta is an effective follicular stimulant, it was concluded by the French Haute Autorité de Santé to provide no clinical added value compared with the long-established comparator product follitropin alfa[46].

There are also other companies (Glycotope GmbH, Berlin, Germany) active at the time of writing working on the development of yet another injectable FSH (FSH-GEX; follitropin epsilon), which also has different pharmacodynamic properties from follitropin alfa. Follitropin epsilon has undergone phase I and II trials[47]. Glycotope is currently seeking development and commercialization partners for a number of its pipeline products; one of which is FSH-GEX and therefore we will have to await further information on the clinical utility of this molecule.

The Introduction of Orally Active GnRH Analogs and Gonadotrophin Receptor Agonists

The "holy grail" of fertility drug development research has been to have a generation of orally bioavailable gonadotropin mimetics: how simple it would then be for our patients!

Our knowledge about the receptor-activating sites of gonadotrophin and GnRH analogs has greatly increased, and the search for small, non-peptide molecules that induce signal transduction without binding to the extracellular domains of membrane proteins has been ongoing for over 20 years. A standard approach has been to use high-throughput screening using cell-based assays of large chemical libraries to find small-molecule (<500 Da) agonists of the receptor. In a classic 2000 review article, Millar and colleagues[48] provided a comprehensive snapshot of the development and commercialization of GnRH peptide analogs with agonistic as well as antagonistic properties. A number of these were just becoming commercially available, including the daily subcutaneous GnRH antagonists, still with us today in ART treatment regimens (cetrorelix, ganirelix). Millar and colleagues also presented a first glimpse of what was in the patent pipeline from a number of commercial laboratories and pharmaceutical companies – in particular Abbott and Takeda – the emergence of nonpeptide GnRH antagonists. Eighteen years later, the United States FDA approved for the first time an orally active nonpeptide GnRH antagonist, elagolix. The drug (Orilissa, brought to the market by AbbVie and in cooperation with Neurocrine Biosciences) is approved for the management of moderate severe pain associated with endometriosis. It is estimated that up to 10% of all women may have endometriosis, with an incidence of around 24–50% in women who experience infertility and in more than 20% who have chronic pelvic pain[49]. Endometriosis may be a lifelong problem, and therefore has the potential to seriously disrupt quality of life and cause significant emotional distress. According to one market analyst, elagolix is projected to become a "blockbuster" with projected sales of $1.35 billion USD by 2022[50].

However, not all in the medical community share the enthusiasm for this new introduction, especially at the projected treatment cost (in the United States the manufacturer AbbVie has priced elagolix at around $10 000 USD a year). In a recent mini review entitled "Elagolix for endometriosis: all that glitters is not gold", Vercellini and colleagues[51] concluded that it is currently not clear whether its use will translate into major benefits for women with endometriosis. They argue that elagolix should not be considered differently to existing GnRH agonists currently in the therapeutic armamentarium.

Irrespective of these arguments, the almost three-decade-long research and development leading to a market introduction of the first orally active GnRH antagonist is certainly an important milestone[52]. Only time will tell if this innovation will become widely used in routine clinical practice.

The development and clinical introduction of an orally active gonadotrophin, however, still eludes us. The first scientific report of a bioactive low molecular weight (LMW) gonadotrophin was in 2002[53]. This molecule was described to act as an FSH receptor antagonist, and could be a potential compound for female contraception. Soon after, other researchers reported small-molecule modulators of the FSH receptor [54] and other compounds (thiazolidinones) with a high affinity for the FSH receptor[55].

The chapter author also reported in 2004/5 on our company's research efforts (Serono International) of the quest for an orally bioavailable gonadotrophin mimetic[56,57]. There was a two-pronged approach to the research: one in the discovery of a potential small molecule (a pyrazolyl tyrosineamide), which could activate the (LH) gonadotrophin receptor and the second avenue through research into biochemical pathways controlling ovarian function, and enzymes, which, when inhibited by specific chemical inhibitors, were able to mimic or amplify gonadotrophin actions. The first avenue of research initially yielded some promising results in a male rat model, but early tests failed to demonstrate ovulatory activity in female animals. The second line of research continued to make progress and a review was published by Nataraja and colleagues[58]. There were, however, a number of important lessons learned following years of intensive research efforts; e.g., first, the immortalized cell-based assay used to screen compounds do not necessarily reflect the compound's ability to stimulate follicle development, and second, finding a molecule with a high potency in vitro does not always correlate with best efficacy in vivo.

There was also another promising lead in the search for an LMW compound with nanomolar potency on the LH receptor. Org 43553 is a hydrogen chloride salt of tert-butyl 5-amino- 2-methylthio-4-(3-(2-(morpholin-4-yl)-acetamido)-phenyl)-thieno[2,3-d] -pyrimidine-6-carboxamide, which was synthesized by the Schering Plough Research Institute at that time in Oss, Netherlands (see Figure 3.1).

Van de Lagemaat and colleagues[59] reported on Org 43553, which demonstrated oral bioavailability and ovulation induction in various animal models as well as testosterone stimulation in male rats. This paper describes succinctly the necessary pathway and testing procedures for a novel small molecule, which is first required prior to use in the human. The data presented provided a solid proof of concept of in vivo physiological LH receptor activation. Additionally, the paper refers to first results in a human clinical study[60], which demonstrated ovulation (by transvaginal ultrasound (TVUS) and elevated progesterone levels) following administration of a single dose of 300 mg.

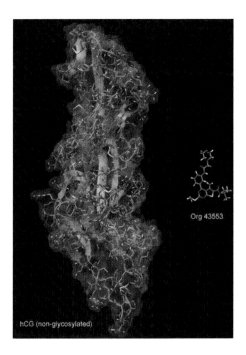

Figure 3.1 X-ray structure of Org 43553: an LMW compound with nanomolar potency on the LH receptor and hCG
Source: van de Lagemaat et al [59]

However, 14 years later, there is still no sign of this novel small molecule coming to the clinic.

The Luteal Phase: Drugs Used and Recent Developments

Following COS in an ART cycle, the luteal phase is markedly different from that in a natural cycle in two important ways. First, since ovarian stimulation produces multiple corpora lutea, the levels of both estradiol (E2) and progesterone (P4) in the early part of the luteal phase are supraphysiologic[61]. Second, and perhaps more important, the duration of ovarian steroid production in COS cycles is usually shorter than normal by 1–3 days. This shortened luteal phase after human menopausal gonadotropin (hMG) use alone has been noted since the earliest days of ART[62].

In view of these various pathologies, luteal phase support (LPS) with P4 or hCG is universally applied in women undergoing ART treatments, particularly if their cycles include the use of GnRH analogs.

The authors of the 2015 Cochrane systematic review[63] concluded that, although the level of evidence was of low quality, both progesterone and hCG administered during the luteal phase are associated with higher rates of live birth or ongoing pregnancy than placebo. Furthermore, P4 supplementation alone resulted in lower rates of OHSS than luteal hCG supplementation. Finally, the route of P4 administration did not appear to be associated with any difference in outcomes, although it could be argued that, because of the supraphysiological endogenous P4 levels present, this may blur any subtle differences between routes and doses of P4 utilized. A recent global survey examining LPS practices (with data from 437 ART clinics) was recently conducted by IVF Worldwide and presented at a congress in Israel[64]. The 3 top treatments of choice for progesterone administration were through vaginal delivery (71%), combination of drugs (12.6%), and intramuscular progesterone (7%). Oral progesterone scored just 1.3%. Of the vaginally delivered progesterones, the most preferred form was a tablet formulation (47%), with progesterone gel scoring 27%.

In view of changes in stimulation protocols (use of GnRH agonist to trigger final follicular maturation[65]) and the availability of two new phase III RCTs[66,67] on the use of oral dydrogesterone (DYD, Duphaston, Abbott, used widely since the 1960s in various gynecological indications), there is now a renewed research focus on LPS regimens.

An individual patient data analysis was carried out using the data from the two phase III studies[68]. There were a total of 1957 patients in the full analysis sample of the two RCTs[66,67] comparing DYD once daily to micronized vaginal progesterone (MVP). The key outcome measures were pregnancy rate at 12 weeks of gestation, live birth rate, and incidence of adverse events of the fetus or newborn (see Table 3.3).

The administration of DYD versus MVP was associated with an increased likelihood of pregnancy at 12 weeks of gestation (OR=1.3, 95% CI: 1.1–1.6; p <0.05) and an increased likelihood of a live birth (OR=1.3, 95% CI: 1.0–1.6; p <0.05). No significant impact of treatment could be found regarding the incidence of "congenital, familial, and genetic disorders" adverse events[68].

Additionally, there is today a reemerging focus on the efficacy of current LPS regimens[69,70]. In view of other recent investigator trials questioning the efficacy of recommended vaginal P4 dose regimens[71] and the widespread preference of patients for oral compounds, there is a call for dydrogesterone to be considered as the new standard in fresh ET cycles[72].

Finally, in terms of innovative new drugs for improving implantation during the early stages of the luteal phase there have been some very encouraging clinical data for an oral oxytocin receptor antagonist (Nolasiban, ObsEva, Geneva, Switzerland). ObsEva licensed nolasiban from Merck KGaA, Darmstadt, Germany, in 2013 and retains worldwide, exclusive, commercial rights.

Nolasiban has the potential to decrease uterine contractions and improve uterine blood flow. Visnova and colleagues[73] recently reported the results of the IMPLANT 2 phase III IVF clinical data of nolasiban administered as a single, 900 mg oral dose 4 hours before either day 3 or 5 fresh single-ET. The primary endpoint results of IMPLANT 2 showed an improvement in the rate of ongoing pregnancy 10 weeks post either day 3 or day 5 ET, with nolasiban treatment versus placebo, 35.6% versus 28.5% (p=0.031), a 25% increase. For women undergoing day 5 ET, nolasiban resulted in an OPR of 45.9% versus 34.7% for placebo (p=0.034): a 32% increase. Live birth rates were also significantly higher (p=0.025) for both cleavage embryo and blastocyst transfer following nolasiban. The safety and tolerability of nolasiban was comparable to placebo, with no increase in serious adverse events, ectopic pregnancy, or congenital birth defects.

A multinational RCT of nolasiban 900 mg in women undergoing IVF (IMPLANT 4) started in November 2018.

Table 3.3 Individual patient data analysis from two phase III studies comparing DYD once daily to MVP

Category	Oral DYD (n=991)	MVP (n=966)	Total (n=1957)
Mean age years (SD)	32.2 (4.5)	32.1 (4.5)	32.2 (4.5)
%<35 years	67	67	67
%>35 years	33	33	33
Mean BMI, kg/m^2 (SD)	23.3 (3.2)	23.2 (3.0)	23.2 (3.1)

Results of Logistic regression	Oral DYD (rate per 1000 women)	MVP (rate per 1000 women)	Odds ratio (DVD vs MVP)	95% CI	P value
Ongoing pregnancy (12 weeks)	381	341	1.32	1.08, 1.61	<0.05
Live birth	344	312	1.28	1.04, 1.56	<0.05

Source: Griesinger, Blockeel, Kahler & Pexman-Fieth, ASRM, 2018 Denver

Summary and Concluding Remarks

The incredible growth and development of the ART field is a remarkable story. The field has led to the development of a number of other treatments, which have expanded the utility of ART, such as use of donor eggs, ICSI, oocyte vitrification, and important, risk-identifying screening technologies. Also, around the IVF laboratory there has been an explosion in gamete research and the development of numerous medical devices.

As far as drug use goes, COS will remain a core foundation stone of any ART treatment especially following recent study findings (importance of number of oocytes collected) and protocol changes (use of freeze-all strategies, vitrification technology, and cumulative live birth data originating from one cycle of ovarian stimulation). Tremendous progress has been made from the introduction of recombinant gonadotrophins in terms of drug quality, consistency[74], and use of pen delivery devices. However, as far as the development and introduction of radically different drug classes to supersede gonadotrophins, two decades of research have proved to be futile.

Some of the reasons were explored in this chapter: the risks of drug development versus return in an area where the number of ART treatments worldwide is relatively small, and different regulatory requirements for registration in main markets, are just a couple. However, important advancements have been made as far as GnRH analogs are concerned, with orally active antagonists available but in a therapeutic area requiring long-term treatment. There could be a major preference change in the type of progesterone used with the availability of further clinical data for oral dydrogesterone.

References

1. Elder K, Johnson MH. The Oldham Notebooks: An Analysis of the Development of IVF 1969–1978. I. Introduction, Materials and Methods. *Reprod Biomed Soc Online.* 2015; 1(**1**): 3–8.

2. Elder K, Johnson MH. The Oldham Notebooks: An Analysis of the Development of IVF 1969–1978. II. The Treatment Cycles and Their Outcomes. *Reprod Biomed Soc Online.* 2015; 1(**1**): 9–18.

3. Steptoe PC, Edwards RG. Reimplantation of a Human Embryo with Subsequent Tubal Pregnancy. *Lancet.* 1976; 1(**7965**): 880–2.

4. Steptoe PC, Edwards RG. Birth After the Reimplantation of a Human Embryo. *Lancet.* 1978; 2(**8085**): 366.

5. Cohen J, Trounson A, Dawson K, et al. The Early Days of IVF Outside the UK. *Hum Reprod Update.* 2005; 11(**5**): 439–59.

6. Edwards RG, Lobo R, Bouchard P. Time to Revolutionize Ovarian Stimulation. *Hum Reprod.* 1996; 11(**5**): 917–19.

7. Alper MM, Fauser BC Ovarian Stimulation Protocols for IVF: Is More Better Than Less? *Reprod Biomed Online.* 2017; 34(**4**): 345–53.

8. Drakopoulos P, Blockeel C, Stoop D, et al. Conventional Ovarian Stimulation and Single Embryo Transfer for IVF/ICSI. How Many Oocytes Do We Need to Maximize Cumulative Live Birth Rates After Utilization of All Fresh and Frozen Embryos? *Hum Reprod.* 2016; 31(**2**): 370–6.

9. Polyzos NP, Drakopoulos P, Parra J, et al. Cumulative Live Birth Rates According to the Number of Oocytes Retrieved After the First Ovarian Stimulation for in Vitro Fertilization/Intracytoplasmic Sperm Injection: A Multicenter Multinational Analysis Including ~15,000 Women. *Fertil Steril.* 2018; 110(**4**): 661–70.

10. Howles CM. Genetic Engineering of Human FSH (Gonal-F). *Hum Reprod Update.* 1996; 2: 172–91.

11. Ludwig M, Felberbaum RE, Diedrich K, Lunenfeld B. Ovarian Stimulation: From Basic Science to Clinical Application. *Reprod Biomed Online.* 2002; 5 Suppl 1: 73–86.

12. Lunenfeld B. Historical Perspectives in Gonadotrophin Therapy. *Hum Reprod Update.* 2004; 10: 453–67.

13. DiMasi JA. Assessing Pharmaceutical Research and Development Costs. *JAMA Intern Med.* 2018; 178(**4**): 587.

14. Howles CM. The Development of Ovarian Stimulation for IVF in in-Vitro Fertilisation: The Pioneers' History. In: Kovacs G, Brinsden P. (eds.). UK: Cambridge University Press. 2018; 202–7.

15. Kushnir VA, Barad DH, Albertini DF, Darmon SK, Gleicher N. Systematic Review of Worldwide Trends in Assisted Reproductive Technology 2004–2013. *Reprod Biol Endocrinol.* 2017; 15(**1**): 6.

16. ESHRE conference. (2018) ICMART report. Online article. www .sciencedaily.com/releases/2018/07/18070 3084127.htm

17. Howles CM, Saunders H, Alam V, Engrand P. FSH Treatment Guidelines Clinical Panel. Predictive Factors and a Corresponding Treatment Algorithm for Controlled Ovarian Stimulation in Patients Treated with Recombinant Human Follicle Stimulating Hormone (Follitropin Alfa) During Assisted Reproduction Technology (ART) Procedures. An Analysis of 1378 Patients. *Curr Med Res Opin.* 2006.

18. DiMasi JA, Grabowski HG, Hansen RW. Innovation in the Pharmaceutical Industry: New Estimates of R&D Costs. *J Health Econ.* 2016; 47: 20–33.

19. Office of Health Economics. The R&D Cost of a New Medicine. Online article. www.ohe.org/publications/rd-cost-new-medicine

20. Agrawal R, West C, Conway GS, Page ML, Jacobs, HS. Pregnancy After Treatment with Three Recombinant Gonadotropins. *Lancet.* 1997; 349: 29–30.

21. Humaidan P, Chin W, Rogoff D, et al. ESPART Study Investigators. Efficacy and Safety of Follitropin Alfa/Lutropin Alfa in ART: A Randomized Controlled Trial in Poor Ovarian Responders. *Hum Reprod.* 2017; 32(**3**): 544–55.

22. de Mora F, Fauser BCJM. Biosimilars to Recombinant Human FSH Medicines: Comparable Efficacy and Safety to the Original Biologic. *Reprod Biomed Online.* 2017;35(**1**): 81–6.

23. FDA Questions & Answers on Biosimilar Development. (2018). Online article. www .fda.gov/downloads/drugs/guidances/uc m444661.pdf

24. Blackstone and Fuhr Joseph. (2013). Let's See How Biosimilars Are Developed. Online article. www.pfizerbiosimilars.com /biosimilars-development

25. Howles CM, Loumaye E, Giroud D, Luyet G. Multiple Follicular Development and Ovarian Steroidogenesis Following Subcutaneous Administration of a Highly Purified Urinary FSH Preparation in Pituitary Desensitized Women Undergoing IVF: A Multicentre European Phase III Study. *Hum Reprod.* 1994; 9(**3**): 424–30.

26. Quintans CJ, Donaldson MJ, Blanco LA, Pasqualini RS. Empty Follicle Syndrome Due to Human Errors: Its Occurrence in an in-Vitro Fertilization Programme. *Hum Reprod.* 1998; 13(**10**): 2703–5.

27. Markle RL, King PJ, Martin DB. Characteristics of a Successful Human Chorionic Gonadotropin (hCG) Administration in Assisted Reproduction. *Fertil Steril.* 2002; 78(Suppl 1): S71–2.

28. Snaifer E, Hugues JN, Poncelet C, Sifer C, Pasquier M, Cedrin-Durnerin I. "Empty Follicle Syndrome" After Human Error: Pregnancy Obtained After Repeated Oocyte Retrieval in a Gonadotropin-Releasing Hormone Antagonist Cycle. *Fertil Steril.* 2008; 90 (**3**): 850.e13–15.

29. Weiss N. Gonadotrophin Products: Empowering Patients to Choose the Product That Meets Their Needs. *Reprod Biomed Online.* 2007; 15: 31–7.

30. Saunders H, de la Fuente Bitaine L, Eftekhar C, et al. Functionality of a Novel Follitropin Alfa Pen Injector: Results from Human Factor Interactions by Patients and Nurses. *Expert Opin Drug Deliv.* 2018; 15(**6**): 549–58.

31. Zitoun P, Parikh J, Nijs M, Zhang W, Levy-Toledano R. Tang B. Analysis of Patient and Nurse Preferences for Self-Administered FSH Injection Devices in Select European Markets. *Int J Womens Health.* 2019; 11: 11–21.

32. Sedbon E, Wainer R, Perves C. Quality of Life of Patients Undergoing Ovarian Stimulation with Injectable Drugs in Relation to Medical Practice in France. *Reprod Biomed Online.* 2006; 12, 298–303.

33. Huisman D, Raymakers X, Hoomans EH. Understanding the Burden of Ovarian Stimulation: Fertility Expert and Patient Perceptions. *Reprod Biomed Online.* 2009; 19 Suppl 2: 5–10.

34. Verberg MF, Eijkemans MJ, Heijnen EM, et al. Why Do Couples Drop-out from IVF Treatment? A Prospective Cohort Study. *Hum Reprod.* 2008; 23(**9**): 2050–5.

35. Brod M, Verhaak CM, Wiebinga CJ, Gerris J, Hoomans EH. Improving Clinical Understanding of the Effect of Ovarian Stimulation on Women's Lives. *Reprod Biomed Online.* 2009; 18(**3**): 391–400.

36. Fares FA, Suganuma N, Nishimori K, et al. Design of a Long-Acting Follitropin Agonist by Fusing the C-Terminal Sequence of the Chorionic Gonadotropin Beta Subunit to the Follitropin Beta Subunit. *Proc Natl Acad Sci USA.* 1992; 89: 4304–8.

37. Beckers NG, Macklon NS, Devroey P, Platteau P, Boerrigter PJ, Fauser BC. First Live Birth After Ovarian Stimulation Using a Chimeric Long-Acting Human Recombinant Follicle-Stimulating Hormone (FSH) Agonist (recFSH-CTP) For in Vitro Fertilization. *Fertil Steril.* 2003; 79(**3**): 621–3.

38. Merck & Co Annual Report for the Fiscal Year Ended Dec 31 2015 (filed with the Securities and Exchange Commission in February 2016). Online report. www .sec.gov/Archives/edgar/data/310158/000 031015816000063/mrk1231201510k.htm

39. le Cotonnec JY, Porchet HC, Beltrami V, Khan A, Toon S, Rowland M. Clinical Pharmacology of Recombinant Human

Follicle-Stimulating Hormone (FSH).
I. Comparative pharmacokinetics with
urinary human FSH. *Fertil Steril.* 1994; 61
(**4**): 669–78.

40. Scholtes MC, Schnittert B,
van Hoogstraten D, Verhoeven
HC, Zrener A, Warne DW.
A Comparison of 3-Day and Daily
Follicle-Stimulating Hormone Injections
on Stimulation Days 1–6 in Women
Undergoing Controlled Ovarian
Hyperstimulation. *Fertil Steril.* 2004; 81:
996–1001.

41. Sharma V, Williams J, Collins W,
Riddle A, Mason B, Whitehead M.
A Comparison of Treatments with
Exogenous FSH to Promote
Folliculogenesis in Patients with
Quiescent Ovaries Due to the
Continued Administration of an
LH-RH Agonist. *Hum Reprod.* 1987; 2:
553–6.

42. ClinicalTrials.gov Identifier:
NCT03019575. Efficacy and Safety of
Corifollitropin Alfa (MK-8962) in
Combination With Human Chorionic
Gonadotropin (hCG) in Adolescent Males
With Hypogonadotropic Hypogonadism
(HH). Online article. https://clinicaltrials
.gov/ct2/show/NCT03019575

43. Howles CM, Tanaka T, Matsuda T.
Management of Male Hypogonadotrophic
Hypogonadism. *Endocr J.* 2007; 54(**2**):
177–90.

44. Olsson H, Sandstrom R, Grundemar L.
Different Pharmacokinetic and
Pharmacodynamic Properties of
Recombinant Follicle-Stimulating
Hormone (rFSH) Derived from a Human
Cell Line Compared with rFSH from a
Non-Human Cell Line. *J Clin Pharmacol.*
2014; 54: 1299–307.

45. Arce JC, Andersen AN, Fernández-
Sánchez M, et al. Ovarian Response
to Recombinant Human Follicle-
Stimulating Hormone: A Randomized,
Antimüllerian Hormone-Stratified,
Dose-Response Trial in Women
Undergoing in Vitro Fertilization/
Intracytoplasmic Sperm Injection.
Fertil Steril. 2014; 102: 1633–40.

46. Haute Autorité de Santé. Online article.
https://www.has-sante.fr/upload/docs/appl
ication/pdf/2017-09/rekovelle_summary
_ct15912.pdf

47. Abd-Elaziz K, Duijkers I, Stöckl L, et al.
A New Fully Human Recombinant FSH
(Follitropin Epsilon): Two Phase
I Randomized Placebo and
Comparator-Controlled Pharmacokinetic
and Pharmacodynamic Trials. *Hum
Reprod.* 2017; 7: 1–9.

48. Millar RP, Zhu YF, Chen C, Struthers RS.
Progress Towards the Development of
Non-Peptide Orally-Active
Gonadotropin-Releasing Hormone (GnRH)
Antagonists: Therapeutic Implications. *Br
Med Bull.* 2000; 56(3): 761–72.

49. ASRM fact sheet Endometriosis. Online
article. www.reproductivefacts.org/news-
and-publications/patient-fact-sheets-and-
booklets/documents/fact-sheets-and-info
-booklets/endometriosis-booklet

50. Clarivate Analytics. (2018). Sales Forecasts
Rise for AbbVie's Elagolix Following
Expected Approval in Endometriosis.
Online article. https://clarivate.com/blog/
life-sciences-connect/sales-forecasts-rise-
for-abbvies-elagolix-following-expected-
approval-in-endometriosis/

51. Vercellini P, Viganò P, Barbara G,
Buggio L, Somigliana E. "Luigi
Mangiagalli" Endometriosis Study Group.
Elagolix for Endometriosis: All That
Glitters Is Not Gold. *Hum Reprod.* 2018.

52. Paulson RJ. At Last, an Orally Active
Gonadotropin-Releasing Hormone
Antagonist. *Fertil Steril.* 2019; 111(**1**): 30–1.

53. Arey BJ, Deecher DC, Shen ES, et al.
Identification and Characterization of
a Selective, Nonpeptide Follicle-
Stimulating Hormone Receptor
Antagonist. *Endocrinology.* 2002; 143.

54. Guo T, Adang AE, Dolle RE, et al. Small
Molecule Biaryl FSH Receptor Agonists.
Part 1: Lead Discovery Via Encoded
Combinatorial Synthesis. *Bioorg Med
Chem Lett.* 2004; 14(7): 1713–16.

55. Maclean D, Holden F, Davis AM, et al.
Agonists of the Follicle Stimulating
Hormone Receptor from an Encoded

Thiazolidinone Library. *J Comb Chem*. 2004; 6.

56. Howles CM, Arkinstall S. Developing new therapeutics for ART: recombinant DNA technology and beyond. In: *Textbook of Assisted Reproductive Techniques: Laboratory and Clinical Perspectives Edition: 1*. Gardner DK, Weissman A, Howles CM, Shoham Z (eds.). Taylor & Francis.

57. Palmer SS, McKenna S, Arkinstall S. Discovery of New Molecules for Future Treatment of Infertility. *Reprod Biomed Online*. 2005; 10 Suppl 3: 45–54.

58. Nataraja SG, Yu HN, Palmer SS. Discovery and Development of Small Molecule Allosteric Modulators of Glycoprotein Hormone Receptors. *Front Endocrinol (Lausanne)*. 2015; 6: 142.

59. van de Lagemaat R, Timmers CM, Kelder J, van Koppen C, Mosselman S, Hanssen RG. Induction of Ovulation by a Potent, Orally Active, Low Molecular Weight Agonist (Org 43553) of the Luteinizing Hormone Receptor. *Hum Reprod*. 2009; 24(**3**): 640–8.

60. Mannaerts B. Novel FSH and LH agonists. From anovulation to assisted reproduction. Proceedings of the Fourth World Congress on Ovulation. In: Filicori M (ed.) 2004; 157–72.

61. Howles CM, Macnamee MC, Edwards RG. Follicular Development and Early Luteal Function of Conception and Non-Conceptional Cycles After Human in-Vitro Fertilization: Endocrine Correlates. *Hum Reprod*. 1987; 2(**1**): 17–21.

62. Jones HW, Jr., Jones GS, Andrews MC, et al. The Program for in Vitro Fertilization at Norfolk. *Fertil Steril* 1982; **38**: 14–21.

63. van der Linden M, Buckingham K, Farquhar C, Kremer JA, Metwally M. Luteal Phase Support for Assisted Reproduction Cycles. *Cochrane Database Syst Rev*. 2015; CD009154.

64. Weissman A. A Survey on Luteal-Phase Support. (2018). ISARG Conference, Tel Aviv, Israel. Online article. http://cme-utilities.com/mailshotcme/SARG/Presentations/1200_Weissman_B_Tue.pdf

65. Humaidan P, Bredkjaer HE, Bungum L, et al. GnRH Agonist (Buserelin) or hCG for Ovulation Induction in GnRH Antagonist IVF/ICSI Cycles: A Prospective Randomized Study. *Hum Reprod*. 2005; 20: 1213–20.

66. Tournaye H, Sukhikh GT, Kahler E, Griesinger G. A Phase III Randomized Controlled Trial Comparing the Efficacy, Safety and Tolerability of Oral Dydrogesterone Versus Micronized Vaginal Progesterone for Luteal Support in in Vitro Fertilization. *Hum Reprod*. 2017; 32(**10**): 2152.

67. Griesinger G, Blockeel C, Sukhikh GT, et al. Oral Dydrogesterone Versus Intravaginal Micronized Progesterone Gel for Luteal Phase Support in IVF: A Randomized Clinical Trial. *Hum Reprod*. 2018; 33(**12**): 2212–21.

68. Griesinger G, Blockeel C, Kahler E, Pexman-Fieth C. Use of Oral Dydrogesterone for Luteal Phase Support in Fresh IVF Cycles Is Associated with an Increase in Live Birth Rate: An Integrated Individual Patient Data Analysis of the Lotus Phase III Trial Program. *Fertil Steril*. 2018; 110(**4**): e90.

69. Labarta E, Mariani G, Holtmann N, Celada P, Remohí J, Bosch E. Low Serum Progesterone on the Day of Embryo Transfer Is Associated with a Diminished Ongoing Pregnancy Rate in Oocyte Donation Cycles After Artificial Endometrial Preparation: A Prospective Study. *Hum Reprod*. 2017; 32(**12**): 2437–42.

70. Alsbjerg B, Thomsen L, Elbaek HO, et al. Progesterone Levels on Pregnancy Test Day After Hormone Replacement Therapy-Cryopreserved Embryo Transfer Cycles and Related Reproductive Outcomes. *Reprod Biomed Online*. 2018; 37(**5**): 641–7.

71. Alsbjerg B, Polyzos NP, Elbaek HO, Povlsen BB, Andersen CY, Humaidan P. Increasing Vaginal Progesterone Gel Supplementation After Frozen-Thawed Embryo Transfer Significantly Increases

the Delivery Rate. *Reprod Biomed Online.* 2013; 26(**2**): 133–7.

72. Griesinger G, Blockeel C, Tournaye H. Oral Dydrogesterone for Luteal Phase Support in Fresh in Vitro Fertilization Cycles: A New Standard? *Fertil Steril.* 2018; 109(**5**): 756–62.

73. Visnova H, Tournaye H, Humberstone A, Terrill P, Macgregor L, Loumaye E. A Placebo-Controlled, Randomized, Double-Blind, Phase 3 Study Assessing Ongoing Pregnancy Rates After Single Oral Administration of a Novel Oxytocin Receptor Antagonist, Nolasiban, Prior to Single Embryo Transfer. *Fertil Steril.* 2018; 110(**4**): e45.

74. Howles CM. Recombinant Gonadotrophins in Reproductive Medicine: The Gold Standard of Today. *Reprod Biomed Online.* 2006; 12: 11–13.

ART Monitoring: An End to Frequent Clinic Visits and Needle Sticks?

Jan Gerris

Introduction

Since the early eighties there has been tremendous evolution in the clinical approach to ART and in how to practically carry execution of these treatments. From a patients' perspective, some of the most significant innovations were: complete replacement of laparoscopic oocyte retrieval under general anesthesia by transvaginal puncture guided by sonography; total disappearance of E2 monitoring using urinary assessments in favor of serum determinations; clinical use of both agonists and antagonists to suppress endogenous LH-peaks avoiding LH-peak monitoring through three-hourly urine collections; specifically designed calibrated devices, called pens, to allow patients to inject daily gonadotrophins themselves instead of being dependent on nurses or hospital facilities willing to inject hCG at odd hours; and recognition of psychological stress leading to active intervention of mental-health professionals in helping patients to cope with both the infertility and with its treatments. Other developments of a more technical nature have widened and optimized treatments – e.g., the successful introduction of ICSI, surgical testicular sperm extraction techniques, preimplantation genetic diagnosis and of blastocyst culture – or have drastically reduced the most frequent complications of ART; i.e., multiple pregnancies (by judicious application of single ET) and OHSS. All these and some other, perhaps minor, improvements have been reported by patients themselves as very welcome developments indeed.

Other innovations with an uncertain future have to find proper indications for their use; e.g., volumetric sonographic assessment of follicular growth, PGT, intravaginal embryo culture, time-lapse aided embryo selection, endometrial implantation assessment, sperm DNA-fragmentation measurement, and others; although these tend to be more of an improvement at the care providers' side than at the patients' side. Generally speaking, one can say that ART has reached clinical maturity thanks to a combination of efficacy and safety. But innovations at both sides of the fence are still welcome.

Moreover, in some but far from all countries, access to treatment is facilitated through reimbursement by health insurers, depending on the type of social security system adopted in each country, region, or state. In some areas, up to six IVF attempts in a lifetime are covered; in others just three or four; in most areas unfortunately, the patient pays all associated IVF costs.

All these developments, where they are available, have allowed couples to conduct more attempts and thus continue their treatment until a successful outcome.

Nevertheless, a number of practical challenges remain, at least from the patients' point of view. The vision behind this book states: as clinical and laboratory protocols become more standardized, clinics will seek to maintain competitive advantage by upgrading to the next stage of economic values: by improving customer experiences – the "experience economy." The question to be answered, therefore, is to propose methods of improving the patient experience throughout treatment.

This chapter focuses on two realistic ways to improve the patients' experience of the clinical trajectory that are knocking at the door but have not been let in yet. The chapter discusses how patient-friendly IVF will lessen the intrusion from the arduous process of IVF. In many cases IVF treatment infiltrates into the life of a couple for up to a month because of numerous monitoring visits before and after their egg retrieval and transfer. We discuss two innovations that liberate the couples during this period of treatment: home-based ultrasound and saliva-based hormone testing.

Home Sonography

The Challenge: Frequent Clinic Visits for Ovarian Sonograms

The need for serial vaginal sonographies to monitor ovarian stimulation for ART treatments remains a major logistic challenge for patients as well as for health-care providers. This hampers access to ART treatment for many couples or renders it strenuous and expensive from an organizational point of view (Figure 4.1).

Sonograms are currently made by various care providers: gynecologists, reproductive nurses, midwives, radiologists, sonographers. Traditionally, for monitoring of ovarian stimulation, women have to come to the care provider working at or collaborating with the center. This could include different personnel or the same during a single cycle. A Cochrane review states in plain language that following up the follicular phase of an IVF/ICSI attempt by ultrasound alone yields similar results to ultrasound combined with hormone determinations[1,2], putting sonography at the crux of cycle monitoring.

Recording images using a vaginal probe is in itself an easy procedure, entailing no risks or health hazard. Making a sonogram is technically such a simple and a no-risk gesture that it does not necessarily need to be performed by a health-care professional and certainly not by a highly specialized reproductive physician. The chapter author has explored in a step-wise manner whether self-operated endo-vaginal telemonitoring (SOET), simply called home sonography, could be a method for patients and/or their partners to make vaginal sonographies themselves anytime, anywhere[3–7], assuming this would alleviate the stress of the monitoring period.

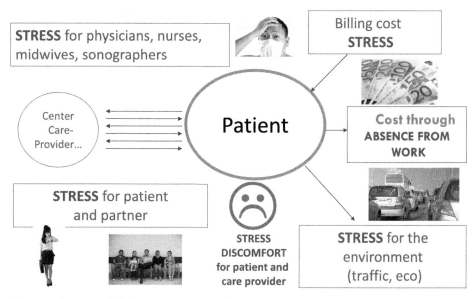

Figure 4.1 The rationale for home monitoring in relation to relieving patient stress

A Practical Solution

Home sonography allows patients to make their sonograms themselves using a small, safe, and easy-to-use customized device, allowing registration of real-time images under direct visual control of the patient or her partner (Figure 4.2). The instrument consists of a tablet PC, to which a vaginal probe is connected using USB technology. Images are sent with proper identification and secured privacy over the Internet to the center where a care provider receives, stores, analyzes, and interprets the images. A structured report is sent, containing advice on the dose of gonadotropins to be self-injected during the following day(s)[8], the timing for the next sonogram, the precise timing of hCG injection, and of oocyte retrieval.

Initially we questioned 25 consecutive couples regarding their attitude toward home sonography. Their willingness to use a SOET technology prompted further research[3].

Then we sought proof of concept. During 20 attempts, patients were monitored traditionally by one physician. After each sonogram, they repeated the sonogram themselves using normal hospital equipment. Images were sent over the hospital intranet as a proxy for the worldwide Internet, stored at the receiving end of a connected in-house PC, and replayed for measurement and analysis. Another physician, blinded to the treatment, later repeated all measurements in one single session. There was excellent congruence between both sets of measurements and a perfect overlap between all clinical decisions taken by both observers. All patients agreed on a very positive experience, as did the midwives involved in this early phase of the study[4].

Next, a two-year prospective randomized trial was conducted comparing clinical and laboratory outcomes between home sonography (using a prototype instrument, now not in use anymore) and traditional sonography, as well as patient-reported outcomes and a health-economic analysis[5]. Inclusion criteria were: <41 years of age, ICSI, no poor

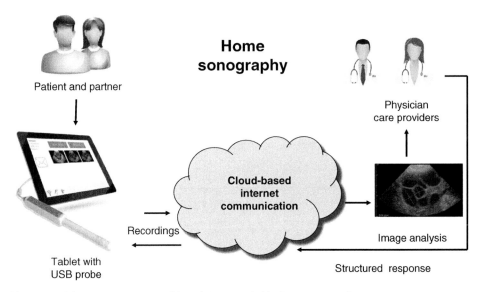

Figure 4.2 Schematic presentation of the solution provided by home sonography

response, two ovaries. One-hundred-and-twenty-one randomized patients completed the study cycle with (n=59) or without (n=62) home sonography. Patient characteristics (age, partner age, BMI, smoking, treatment rank, AMH) in both groups were comparable. Similar conception rates were obtained, as well as a similar number of follicles >15 mm. The number of ova at ovum pickup, (log 2 of) the number of metaphase II oocytes, the number of transferable embryos available at ET, the number of morphologically excellent embryos, and the number of embryos frozen were all comparable. The home sonography group showed a significantly higher feeling of empowerment and more partner participation than the control group. Comparing home sonography patients with their own historical controls in previous attempts, which were monitored traditionally, showed an increased feeling of empowerment, partner participation, feeling of discretion, less stress, and a trend toward more contentedness. A health-economic analysis showed home sonography cycles to have significant financial advantage over traditional monitoring. In particular, the cost of transportation for the patient was lower[5].

Advantages of Home Telemonitoring

A comparison between the disadvantages of the present way of monitoring ovarian stimulation for ART and the advantages of SOET as we have experienced it until today is pictured in Figures 4.1–4.3. Patients do not need to go the center to have sonograms performed. This saves them time and money spent on gas, car usage, train, or bus. They avoid loss of income during working hours. Weekends and their important social and household functions are less interrupted by half- or full-day trips to the center. Patients living far from centers do not have to spend time or money for costly stays of a week or more at a hotel near the center. Centers performing IVF are less crowded by routine

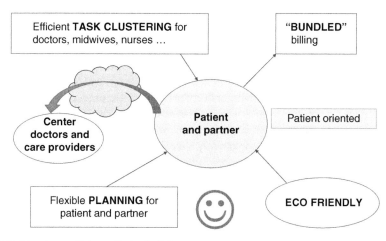

Figure 4.3 Advantages of telemonitoring in ART

patients only needing a sonogram. Measurements based on home sonograms are more standardized and reproducible and can be performed at ease, allowing decreased inter-observer variation.

Communication with the patient is smoother, more complete and more personalized, and all information needed is documented in print. Questions accompanying the images are answered properly and not hurriedly by a stressed doctor, midwife, or nurse. More time is thus available for truly necessary interactions between doctors/nurses and patients that need to be performed in person with the staff at the center. This reduces excessively long waiting lists for consultations of new patients. Treatments are possible for patients who live far from the center. Home sonography makes follow-up of ovarian stimulation easier not only for the patient but also for the physician as well because images can be retrieved and analyzed at any time and in any place where Wi-Fi is available.

Billing can be simplified by using a fixed price for one monitoring ART ovarian stimulation attempt instead of per sonography, leaving the method used to monitor free to doctor and patient. A major hidden aspect resides at the employers' side or by avoiding loss of direct income and transportation cost in those with independent jobs. There is more convenience and discretion for the patient and a stronger involvement of the partner, now often reduced to the role of driver. The sheer feeling of empowerment in women and their partners is clearly enhanced. Sonograms can also be made or assisted by the partner who, in 50% of cases, is at the origin of the subfertility and, in many cases, will be more than happy to be able to participate in an active way.

Home sonography is not intended to replace all standard sonograms made by professional care providers. These will remain needed in complicated cases, or when abnormal images (e.g., cysts, hydrosalpinges, unexpected tumors, endometriosis) are observed, or at the request from the anxious type of patient. It is meant to *alleviate* an abnormal amount of time-consuming, routine work, and to allow patients living far from the center to make fewer demanding sacrifices.

Present Clinical Experience Using Home Sonography

Following the 2014 RCT, we introduced home sonography as a routine possibility for telemonitoring follicular growth. At present the system is used by a small percentage of patients only.

In one hundred consecutive ICSI cycles in 78 different patients over a 14-month period, the Sonaura system (Sonaura LLC, Fort Collis, Colorado, United States) was used[7]. Patients were counseled regarding the possibility of poor response and hyperstimulation. According to the Cochrane review mentioned earlier, there were no *systematic* serum E2 measurements performed. Patients were shown the introductory movie available at www.mysonaura.com. Teaching is only mandatory in first-time users (n=78), not in repeat users (n=22) because the system is very intuitive, especially for the present generation of young adults raised among tablets and smartphones. For teaching, we use any high-end instrument, either after suppression with an oral contraceptive or early in a natural cycle. The Sonaura system is not presently devised for sonograms during the early follicular phase. A slightly filled bladder may be helpful for teaching, but is not advisable for later recordings. The pelvis should ideally be normal with a normal location of the ovaries. The black streaks of the pulsating iliac artery and the pulseless veins are identified, the adjoining slightly darker grayish ovaries visualized, and, if useful, an antral follicle count is performed. Dilated ovarian veins may be conspicuous. Usually the endometrium is visible, although not with the triple-line image at this time of the cycle. The uterus is outlined as a grayish pear-like organ, containing the endometrium, which will steadily show up as a banana-like figure with a triple-line image. It is also mentioned to the patient that images of the uterus are not very important, because gonadotrophin dosage does not depend on them. A short (15 seconds) registration of the uterus is mainly intended to distinguish left and right ovarian recordings from each other.

Probe movements (sideways, forward, backward, and rotating) are demonstrated when searching for the resting ovaries.

It is always pointed out that home sonography is not a goal in itself, but a facilitating tool. Should either the doctor or the patient desire so, a professional sonogram is possible in the center daily, the full year round. First sonograms are not required before day seven or eight of gonadotropin injection. The patient with the shortest follicular phase received hCG on day nine of stimulation. So-called random stimulation regimens where stimulation is started at any moment of the cycle, are compatible with using Sonaura, for they will more frequently show follicular structure in contrast to day 2–3 or pill-suppressed cycles.

The device used (Figure 4.2) features a patient part and a care provider part. The patient part consists of a dedicated tablet, connectable to an FDA-approved and cost-effectiveness compatible vaginal probe (Interson, Pleasanton, California, United States), delivered in a suitcase with gel, condoms, and written instructions. In between cycles, the probe is sanitized using a specific sporicidal and disinfectant foam (Tristel Duo, Tristel Solutions Limited, UK) based on chlorine dioxide[9,10]. Cleansing within a cycle needs dry cloth or absorptive paper. Images from an ongoing cycle stay on the tablet until it is returned at the time of oocyte retrieval. They are wiped as soon as the cycle is ended by the care provider, which makes the tablet available for another cycle.

Patients perform sonograms at home, but can do so wherever they happen to be if they have access to Wi-Fi. Recordings can be received, analyzed, and responded to by the care provider on different locations as well, all over the world. The idea is to make these interactions fit within the time frame of a regular ART clinic.

Recordings are sent as one uninterrupted recording in a fixed sequence setting: 30 seconds for the right ovary, 15 seconds for the uterus, 30 seconds for the left ovary. Settings are adaptable if wished by the care provider. Recording is started after a search during which the patient sweeps the probe in several directions creating a mental picture of the sequence she intends to record. This takes between 5 and 20 minutes. Women usually scan and record themselves, requiring help from their partners or third parties only if needed. After recording, the patient has access to a communication box where she can write down a message or ask questions.

The care provider part consists of specific software, which can be accessed anytime from any personal computer through a user-specific password. Encrypted and password-protected access to the recordings can be customized per doctor or per center and contains a home page, a list of all patients, a list of patients presently in treatment, and a list of currently active cycles. When creating a new cycle, a cycle-specific password and entry code are generated and automatically sent by email to the patient, who enters them at each recording. The recording is sent to the storage server using an encrypted communication protocol. When a new recording comes in, the care provider is notified by email on his or her mobile phone. For measurement, recordings can be stopped and replayed by the doctor or sonographer as often as needed. All follicles are measured in their two largest perpendicular diameters. After measuring all visible follicles, a reply is entered in the patient communication box comprising a brief description of the stimulation status, dosage instructions, the time when the next sonogram is expected, and, if needed, suggestions to improve image quality or some supportive words. It is then sent to the patient, who is equally notified by email that the response has come in on the tablet. All videos are stored in the cloud from where they can be retrieved again anytime and anywhere; e.g., to compare an ongoing cycle with previous attempts in the same patient. Blockchain technologies may be adapted in the future to add further security to individual patient data.

Patients are instructed to visualize the majority, if not all, of the largest follicles in such a way that the largest diameter and the diameter perpendicular to it come into view at the start of the recording. Recording starts with the probe pointed toward the largest follicle in its largest diameter. This allows the care provider to see immediately if the recording was successful. Almost all patients succeed in making very clear recordings, especially once follicles are >15 mm and nearing the end of stimulation.

Of a total of these 78 different patients, 62 patients went through 1 ICSI attempt using Sonaura, 11 patients went through 2 attempts, 4 patients went through 3 attempts, and 1 patient through 4 attempts. A total of 471 home sonograms were performed and analyzed (mean=4.71±1.48/attempt; range: 2–9). Ninety cycles were conducted without any in situ sonographic control between the start of the treatment and the moment of oocyte retrieval. In ten cycles at least one in situ sonogram was performed. There was only one true method failure; all other cases either confirmed poor or absent follicular growth or were performed for circumstantial reasons.

The total, clinical and OPRs per started cycle were 41%, 36%, and 30%. In 18% of cycles, there was no ET. On a per transfer basis these figures are 48.8%, 42.7%, and 35.4%. There were 30 ongoing pregnancies in 78 different women, equaling 38% of patients who obtained an ongoing pregnancy as of the time of writing. These figures are perfectly comparable to the general figures of the center.

The mean two-way distance per sonogram from home to the center in this series was 376±114 km. With 4.7 sonograms per attempt, this means an average of 1732±698 km of avoided transportation. At €0.3461/km, this is an average saving of €600 per attempt.

There were no complications. The large majority of patients and their partners were very positive about the use of the Sonaura system.

Home Sonography: Conclusion

Although much is published about telemedicine in cardiology, diabetes, and general aspects of telemedicine and e-health, not much has been published with respect to reproductive medicine[11–15]. Experience in the United States with home sonography until today is limited to the group from Boston IVF who reported a limited but carefully conducted pilot study at the 2016 ASRM meeting at Salt Lake City[16].

The system derives its value from two major points: (1) clinical decisions do not differ when taken on the basis of high-end machine sonograms versus on the basis of images made at home by the patient, and (2) complete disjunction between place and time for both patient and care provider, making the process of follow-up very flexible.

Home sonography also increases access to treatment, both in large countries where huge distances have to be covered and in smaller but traffic-jammed countries where access to IVF/ICSI treatment may be a true challenge. This was mainly the case for the patients treated in Belgium, though mostly living in the neighboring Netherlands.

The ideal patient for home sonography is the woman who has already gone through at least one complete ART cycle and is not averse to innovation. She knows what growing follicles look like. She has logistic problems in attending the clinic, or children to attend to, or a very demanding job, or she lives far away. Most patients who have used the system once request to use it again. Though normal responders are easiest to follow, we have used it at their request in known poor responders[17]. She needs to be at ease with a simple vaginal manipulation. Some women are able to send perfect ovarian recordings when follicles are still small, and all find the follicles easily before the largest ones are >15 mm in diameter.

Patients appreciate home sonography not only as a technological innovation but also as a method of improved patient–physician interaction[18].

Though conceived as a method to be used by the patient herself, in some circumstances general practitioners, nurses, midwives, or gynecologists can also be the actual operators of the system sending images to a distant center where the decisions are taken.

The risk for OHSS should not necessarily make patients refrain from using the Sonaura device. Patients are informed that, when OHSS tends to develop, an easy switch can be made toward an all-freeze procedure, in which no embryos are transferred but are all frozen[19]. Regarding image quality, Pereira and colleagues have conducted a study showing a very high correlation between measurements performed subsequently by the patient and by a professional in different clinical situations where follicles were counted and measured[20].

Surely the patient is empowered by being actively involved in her treatment; a fact that strongly determines patient satisfaction. This form of telemedicine can be integrated structurally in how a center works. Actually, interpreting the sonograms is easy to learn and could be conducted by members of the nursing staff, under supervision of reproductive physicians, whose time is thus available for more demanding consultations. Many of these professionals are already engaged in the routine sonographic follow-up in some countries. This fits in a world where telemedicine has already found a firm place in other fields of medicine such as radiology, cardiology, or antenatal home cardiotocography.

In ambitious centers, offering home sonography may help to enlarge their action radius and extend it to distant and thinly populated areas. It can be a distinctive proposal to improve patients' experience. It allows patients to choose the center they prefer because of its reputed high-quality ART laboratory.

Employers are also among the winners as half of the lower cost of home sonography versus traditional monitoring is due to avoiding absence from work[7].

Undoubtedly, like all innovative reproductive technologies, home sonography will also have to stand the test of ethical acceptability[21] and surely further technical improvements can be made to the system.

Other systems based on emerging technology have been introduced; e.g., handheld point-of-care ultrasound (Vscan Connections, General Electric, United States), allowing the physician to gather potentially important sonographic data permitting better patient management and/or referral. However, the idea appears to be that the system is used by a care provider and not by the patient, which is the crux of the Sonaura system.

Although experience is still limited and is expected to remain so for some time because of its disruptive character, home sonography can be a valuable alternative for women undergoing ovarian stimulation for ART. When legal and reimbursement impediments can be dealt with, and once employers and insurers realize that indirect financial gain is possible by making sonograms at home instead of during working hours, it may be a useful alternative for selected patients.

E2 Measurements In Saliva Rather Than In Serum

Introduction

Another perspective for simplification resides in the possibility of replacing serum determinations of E2 by salivary determinations, avoiding the need for venipuncture. Because of the burden for the patient of taking blood samples for E2 assessments, a less invasive alternative would be welcomed.

Monitoring of ovarian stimulation for IVF/ICSI attempts is routinely performed using serum sampling for E2 and ultrasound. Some studies contend that ultrasonography alone is enough. A meta-analysis concluded that monitoring COS by ultrasonography alone is unlikely to cause substantial reduction in the number of oocytes retrieved or alter the chance of achieving a clinical pregnancy. A Cochrane review found similar results and concluded that there is no firm evidence that stimulation monitoring using TVUS alone is less effective or less efficacious than combined monitoring using TVUS and E2 assays, with regard to both clinical pregnancy rates and even the incidence of OHSS. However, the overall quality of the included studies was low. The Cochrane review concluded that a combined monitoring protocol including both TVUS and E2 assay is

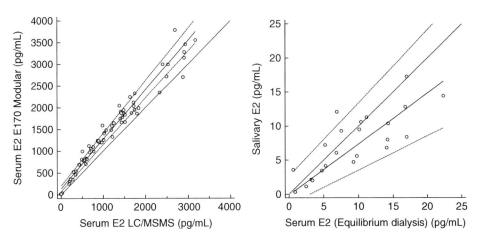

Figure 4.4 Salivary E2 as a surrogate marker for serum E2 in ART: correlation between all values for serum and salivary determinations in ART patients[22]

seen as precautionary good clinical practice and as a confirmatory test in a subset of women to identify those at high risk of OHSS[1,2].

Although monitoring using TVUS and serum E2 is therefore still used as the clinical standard[1], it entails some disadvantages: it is time-intensive and relatively expensive. As it is difficult to predict when patients need to go to clinic due to individually different responses to stimulation, it causes stress for patients as well as for care providers. Some patients have to travel great distances to the nearest hospital. Moreover, phlebotomy is an invasive procedure. We conjectured that it is possible to simplify monitoring of cycles for IVF and ICSI by using saliva sampling instead of serum saliva measurements. Since patients can perform this at home, it could be a time- and cost-saving alternative for phlebotomy. The point-of-care measurement of E2 could be performed either using a micro-drop of blood obtained after puncture at a fingertip or using a passive drool saliva sample, which can be entered into a diagnostic salivary assay kit (e.g., Salimetrix, United States).

Experience with Salivary E2 Measurement

Preliminary studies showed a good clinical correlation between serum and salivary E2 and provide evidence to support the hypothesis that salivary E2 could be used as an indicator for serum E2 (Figures 4.4–4.5)[22–24].

Boston IVF introduced the first needle-free saliva test. Patients can collect their saliva at home in less than five minutes and drop off their samples for analysis each morning [25]. Saliva testing is noninvasive, simple to perform and undergo, safe for the patient and practitioner, stress free, painless, and private and convenient for the patient and his or her physician. Saliva is an excellent medium: because it is a natural ultra-filtrate of blood, it reflects the biologically active (free) fraction of steroids in the bloodstream[26]. Steroid hormones are not bound by carrier proteins. One to ten percent of the steroids in blood leak into saliva from plasma. Albumin and sex hormone-binding globulin do not allow the bound fraction of the hormones to get into saliva due to their molecular weights [26,27].

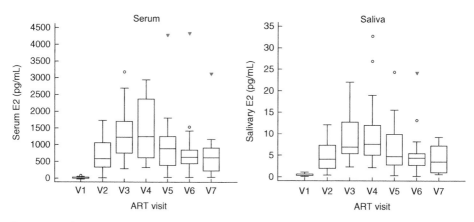

Figure 4.5 Salivary E2 as a surrogate marker for serum E2 in assisted reproduction treatment: parallelism of E2 variation during ART stimulation visits (V) as measured by serum and saliva[22]

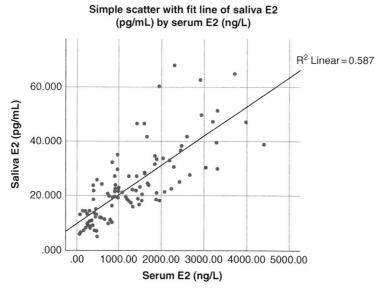

Figure 4.6 Scatter plot showing the linear correlation between levels of serum and saliva E2 during ovarian stimulation for ART[28]

In a recent cooperative study conducted by Boston IVF and Ghent Fertility Centre, a good correlation between serum E2 and the product of the mean diameters of the follicles was found[28] (Figures 4.6–4.9). This is similar to the results of older studies where, in normal menstrual cycles, a good correlation between the diameter of the dominant follicle and the serum E2 concentration was established. It is known that each follicle >18 mm in diameter generates an average of 250–300 pg/mL of the E2 concentration in serum. It is also known for a fact that total follicular volume of both

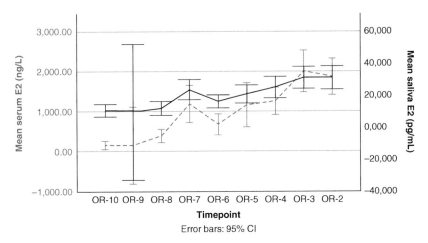

Figure 4.7 Correlation between serum and saliva E2 concentrations during ovarian stimulation for ART. Mean serum E2 (blue, in ng/L) and mean saliva E2 (green, in pg/mL) for all patients with an assessment on that day are both shown on the Y-axis, with confidence interval. The X-axis indicates the time of investigation (OR: oocyte retrieval, n: number of days preceding OR)[28].

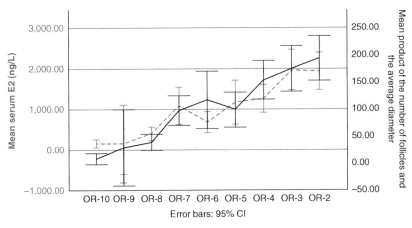

Figure 4.8 Correlation between (a) serum and (b) saliva E2 and the mean of the product of the total number of follicles seen at sonography with their average diameter. The Y-axis shows the mean (a) serum or (b) saliva E2 for all patients who had an investigation on that day and the measurements of the follicles, expressed by the mean product of the number of follicles with their average diameter. The X-axis shows the time of investigation[28]

ovaries and the total follicular volume of the ovary containing the dominant follicle are positively correlated with preovulatory serum E2 levels.

More recent research confirms the good correlation between saliva E2 and serum E2, found in the preliminary studies quoted above. The levels of E2 in serum and saliva increase in a day-to-day manner from the start of stimulation until day two of oocyte retrieval. A high level of serum E2 is associated with a high level of saliva E2. Celec and

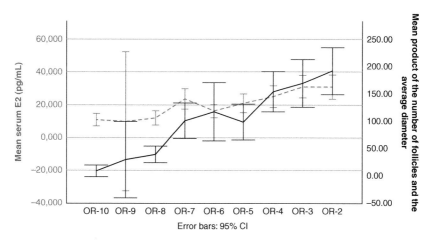

Figure 4.9 Correlation between saliva E2 and the mean of the product of the total number of follicles seen at sonography with their average diameter. The Y-axis shows the mean saliva E2 for all patients who had an investigation on that day and the measurements of the follicles, expressed by the mean product of the number of follicles with their average diameter. The X-axis shows the time of investigation[28].

colleagues found a correlation between salivary and plasma levels in the menstrual cycle [27]. Our findings are similar to previous findings. Alper and colleagues found a good correlation between saliva and serum E2, with a correlation coefficient of 0.88[24]. The authors concluded that saliva E2 is a good surrogate for free E2 in women undergoing COS. Patient survey results showed that saliva sampling was the preferred method of analysis, associated with less anxiety and more likely to be recommended to friends[29].

In our own experience, performed in ART attempts, both serum and saliva E2 correlated with the total number of follicles >10 mm. We conclude that estrogen levels correlate with the total number of developing follicles. During stimulation, follicles develop in an asynchronous manner. Not all follicles become mature. So E2 in saliva and serum correlates with the total number of developing follicles rather than with the number of mature follicles observed on ultrasound.

Salivary E2 Measurements: Conclusion

Serum E2 as well as saliva E2 correlate with sonographically measured follicle growth. Therefore, saliva E2 is a good alternative for serum E2 in monitoring ART cycles. This could simplify the follow-up of ovarian stimulation.

A difficult side of using saliva resides in the preanalytic sample quality. Spitting has to be avoided to avoid clots. Blood contamination due to brushing can make the sample unusable. In blood-contaminated samples, salivary E2 values are elevated. This can adversely influence clinical interpretations.

The big advantage of saliva measurement is that saliva can be produced at home. In remote areas, in our stressful, busy lives, the patient can produce saliva in her own free time and put it in a postbox at a convenient moment[24]. The development of a semiquantitative point-of-care test that can also be conducted at home would be the ultimate goal of this technology.

The optimal method of monitoring ovarian stimulation in IVF/ICSI cycles remains to be debated. The Cochrane study published in 2014 concludes that a combination of ultrasound and E2 may need to be retained as good clinical practice and as a confirmatory test for those at risk for OHSS. A strong correlation between saliva and serum E2 was found by several investigators. Moreover, both correlate well with the product of the number of follicles and the average diameter, measured with sonography. Salivary E2 measurement is a viable alternative for serum E2. In the larger picture of patient-friendly follow-up of ovulation, salivary sampling can be used not only for ART monitoring but also for non-IVF monitoring of ovulation stimulation as well[7].

In conclusion, given time to gather more clinical data and experience, it is feasible at the time of writing to simplify ovarian stimulation monitoring by replacing on-site visits by home sonograms and it should be within reach to replace blood measurement of E2 by either a point-of-care microdrop blood assay or a salivary measurement. These simple modifications can truly simplify the patient experience during a stressful IVF cycle.

References

1. Kwan I, Bhattacharya S, Kang A, Woolner A. Monitoring of Stimulated Cycles in Assisted Reproduction (IVF and ICSI) (Review). Cochrane Menstrual Disorders and Subfertility Group. 2014.

2. Martins WP, Vieira CV, Teixeira DM, Barbosa MA, Dassunção LA, Nastri CO. Ultrasound for Monitoring Controlled Ovarian Stimulation: A Systematic Review and Meta-Analysis of Randomized Controlled Trials. *Ultrasound Obstet Gynecol.* 2014; 43: 25–33.

3. Gerris J, Geril A, De Sutter P. Patient Acceptance of Self-Operated Endo-Vaginal Tele-Monitoring (SOET): A Step Towards More Patient Friendly ART? *Facts, Views and Vision in Ob/Gyn.* 2009; 1: 161–70.

4. Gerris J, De Sutter P Self-Operated Endo-Vaginal Tele-Monitoring (SOET): A Step Towards More Patient-Centered ART? *Hum Reprod.* 2010; 25: 562–8.

5. Gerris J, Delvigne A, Dhont N et al. Self-Operated Endo-Vaginal Tele-Monitoring Versus Traditional Monitoring of Ovarian Stimulation in Assisted Reproduction: An RCT. *Hum Reprod.* 2014; 29: 1941–8.

6. Gerris J. Self-Operated Endo-Vaginal Tele-Monitoring: Using Internet-Based Home Monitoring of Follicular Growth in Assisted Reproduction Technology. In: *Ultrasonography in Gynecology.* Botros RMB Rizk, Puscheck EE (eds.)

Cambridge University Press. 2015; 369–74.

7. Gerris J, Vandekerckhove F, De Sutter P. Outcome of One Hundred Consecutive ICSI Attempts Using Patient Operated Home Sonography for Monitoring Follicular Growth. *Facts, Views and Vision in Ob/Gyn.* 2016; 141–6.

8. Chen Y, Zhang Y, Hu M et al. Timing of Human Chorionic Gonadotropin (hCG) Hormone Administration in IVF/ICSI Protocols Using GnRH Agonist and Antagonists: A Systematic Review and Meta-Analysis. *Gynecol Endocrinol.* 2014; 30: 431–7.

9. Casalegno J-S, Le Bail Carval K, Eibach D et al. High Risk HPV Contamination of Endo-cavity Vaginal Ultrasound Probes: An Underestimated Route of Nosocomial Infection? *PLoS ONE.* 2012.

10. Ma STC, Yeung AC, Chan PKS et al. Trans-Vaginal Ultrasound Probe Contamination by the Human Papillomavirus in the Emergency Department. *Emerg Med J.* 2012.

11. Agha Z, Schapira M, Laud PW et al. Patient Satisfaction with Physician–Patient Communication During Telemedicine. In: *Telemedicine and e-Health.* Mary Ann Liebert, Inc. 2009; 831–9.

12. Davis RM, Hitch AD, Salaam MM et al. TeleHealth Improves Diabetes Self-Management in an Underserved

Community. *Diabetes Care*. 2010; 33: 1712–7.

13. Khader YS, Jarrah MI, Al-Shudifat AE et al. Telecardiology Application in Jordan: Its Impact on Diagnosis and Disease Management, Patients' Quality of Life, and Time- and Cost-Savings. *Int J Telemed Appl*. 2014.

14. Ferreira AC, O'Mahony E, Hélio A et al. Teleultrasound: Historical Perspective and Clinical Application. *Int J Telemed App*. 2015.

15. Rashid L, Bashshur RL, Shannon GW, Smith BR et al. The Empirical Evidence for the Telemedicine Intervention in Diabetes Management. In: *Telemedicine and e-Health*. Mary Ann Liebert, Inc. 2015; 1–34.

16. Resetkova N, Sakkas D, Bayer S, Penzias A, Alper M. Home Based Ultrasound Monitoring Is a Feasible Method of in Cycle Monitoring. Oral Presentation at ASRM in Salt Lake City, Utah. 2016.

17. Ferraretti AP, La Marca A, Fauser BCJM et al. ESHRE Consensus on the Definition of "Poor Response" to Ovarian Stimulation for *in Vitro* Fertilization: The Bologna Criteria. *Hum Reprod*. 2011; 26: 1616–24.

18. Verdonckt S, Gerris J. Patients' Ideas, Expectations and Experience with Self-Operated Endo-Vaginal Tele-Monitoring: A Prospective Pilot Study. *Facts Views and Vis ObGyn*. 2017.

19. D'Angelo A, Amso NN. Embryo Freezing for Preventing Ovarian Hyperstimulation Syndrome: A Cochrane Review. *Hum Reprod*. 2002; 17: 2787.

20. Pereira I, von Horn K, Depenbusch M et al. Clinical Evaluation of Self-operated Endo-vaginal Tele-monitoring. *Fertil Steril*. 2016.

21. Dondorp W, de Wert G. Innovative Reproductive Technologies: Risks and Responsibilities. *Hum Reprod* 2011; 26: 1604–8.

22. Fiers T, Dielen C, Somers S, Kaufman JM, Gerris J. Salivary Estradiol as a Surrogate Marker for Serum Estradiol in Assisted Reproduction Treatment. *Clin Biochem*. 2017; 50: 145–9.

23. Dielen C, Fiers T, Somers S, Deschepper E, Gerris J. Correlation Between Saliva and Serum Concentrations of E2 in Women Undergoing Ovarian Hyperstimulation with Gonadotropins for IVF/ICSI. *Facts Views Vis Obgyn*. 2017; 9: 85–91.

24. Alper M, Matin M, French B, Widra E, Copperman A, Levy M et al. Blind Validation of Estrogen Monitoring in Controlled Ovarian Stimulation IVF Cycles Using a "Patient-Friendly" Saliva Based E2 Assay. Poster *Am Soc Reprod Med*. 2017 Scientific Congress, Salt Lake City, US.

25. Cision. Boston IVF Pioneers World's First Needle-Free Saliva Test Used in Infertility Treatment; Patient Friendly Monitoring Replaces Daily Blood Tests. Online article. www.prnewswire.com/news-releases/boston-ivf-pioneers-worlds-first-needle-free-saliva-test-used-in-infertility-treatment-patient-friendly-monitoring-replaces-daily-blood-tests-138043113.html

26. Kells J, Dollbaum C. Saliva Test Part 1: Clinical Use, Elements of Testing and Guidelines for Posttreatment Interpretation. *Int J Pharm Comp*. 2009; 13: 280–8.

27. Celec P, Ostatnikova D, Skoknova M, Hodosy J, Putz Z, Kudela M. Salivary Sex Hormones During the Menstrual Cycle. *Endocrine Journal*. 2009; 56: 521–3.

28. Rottiers AS, Dalewyn L, Somers S, Alper MM, Sakkas D, Gerris J. Correlation Between Sonographic Follow-Up of Follicular Growth, Serum Estradiol and Salivary Estradiol in Women Undergoing Controlled Ovarian Stimulation (IVF/ICSI). *Facts Views Vis Obgyn*. 2018; 10(**4**): 173–9.

29. Zimon A, Lannon B, Sheller S, Sakkas D, Ulrich M, Alper M. Venopuncture-Free IVF: Measurement of Estrogen in Controlled Ovarian Stimulation IVF Cycles Using a "Patient-Friendly" Saliva-Based E2 Assay. *ASRM abstracts*. 2013; 100 (3).

The IVF Cycle to Come: Laboratory Innovations

Denny Sakkas and David K Gardner

Introduction

In the first reported case of IVF and embryo development in the human, Rock and Menkin[1,2] made the following description of the culture and development of a fertilized embryo: "The eggs were incubated in serum for 22.5 hours, being washed in salt solution before and after incubation, and then exposed to a washed sperm suspension in Locke's solution[1] for two hours at room temperature. They were again washed in Locke's solution and cultured in fresh serum for 45 hours. When examined at the end of the incubation period, one egg was found to be in the two-cell stage; two blastomeres of fairly uniform size and appearance, and containing granular cytoplasm, were enclosed within a zona pellucida along the border of which were numerous spermatozoa. At least one of them was clearly seen within the zona." Thirty years later, following considerable effort and research, the first IVF birth was described by Steptoe and Edwards in 1978. Many landmarks occurred in the three decades intervening these two reports. In the ensuing 40 years since the birth of Louise Brown, some 70 years after the initial studies of Menkin and Rock, dramatic advances in knowledge and technologies have been made in the IVF laboratory, facilitating live birth rates after transfer to surpass the 50% mark in some patient groups and oocyte donors. The crucial laboratory based advances that have helped these rates to be achieved include ICSI, embryo cryopreservation through vitrification, blastocyst culture, and PGT. What will the next 10–20 years hold and how will the IVF laboratory of the future look?

---

[1] A **solution** isotonic with blood plasma, which contains the chlorides of sodium, potassium, and calcium, and sodium bicarbonate and dextrose, and is used similarly to physiological saline. It is similar to Ringers.

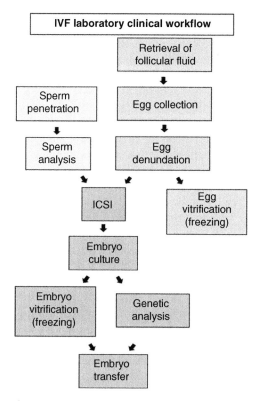

Figure 5.1 Major steps in the current IVF laboratory workflow

The IVF laboratory, the cornerstone of successful IVF, will play an increasingly important role in the coming years in improving live birth rates, but also ensuring that the children born from IVF procedures are healthy and not affected by the procedures themselves[3]. The current laboratory workflow comprises numerous steps (Figure 5.1). This chapter elaborates on the current IVF laboratory workflow and how these steps could be performed in an IVF cycle of the future.

Andrology

Sperm Analysis, Preparation, and Selection

One of the first interfaces of the laboratory with IVF patients is the analysis of the semen sample. Remote analysis of a semen sample has already been described in a number of scenarios. This may be as simple as a sample being sent in a solution to a central laboratory from a patient's home[4] or a patient being able to perform an analysis at home by creating a smartphone video, which will provide information on sperm quality [5]. As will be a consistent theme in the future laboratory, all aspects of the patient's procedure will be accessible through secure access to a patient's individual internet portal (see Chapter 9). This initial semen analysis could provide the basis for the male's future treatment with their partner.

The home-based analysis will provide analysis of sperm concentration, motility, motility patterns, and morphology. A sometimes-forgotten component of semen analysis that may be performed remotely is assessment of oxidative stress. A number of tools are now available to provide further information about semen quality and male infertility. One system, the Male Infertility Oxidative System, is the latest advancement in laboratory assessment of oxidative stress and can establish an oxidative reproductive potential value that is capable of differentiating normal from abnormal semen and fertile from infertile men[6]. Further information on sperm quality, plausibly needed as a marker of child health, will involve molecular analysis of sperm characteristics that should define whether couples will proceed directly to IVF/ICSI or have an equal chance of achieving pregnancy using insemination. Specific methylation and micro RNA profiles of sperm characteristics could be examined to ascertain whether the semen profile of the male will negatively impact success rates. Numerous groups have already shown that the unique nature of the sperm epigenome and the patterns found in mature sperm that appear to reflect perturbations in spermatogenesis may ultimately have an effect on pregnancy outcomes[7–9]. It is believed these traits will provide predictive insight that can be exploited as a diagnostic tool. Indeed, there is emerging data suggesting that the predictive power of DNA methylation and RNA signatures in sperm likely exceeds that which can be found with traditional assessments of male infertility[10–12]. The future andrology laboratory will therefore be equipped with molecular diagnostic capabilities to assess the sperm epigenome as a diagnostic tool in the context of male infertility. Much of the testing will be done in house and analysis likely provided remotely via secure connections.

Sperm preparation will also be performed in a manner that will be aimed at identifying populations of or single sperm that have limited or no risk of passing on paternal traits that could affect fertilization, embryo development, pregnancy, and the health of the offspring. Human epidemiological studies have suggested a relationship between advanced paternal age at conception and adverse neurodevelopmental outcomes in offspring, including an increased risk for psychiatric conditions such as autism and schizophrenia[11]. In a recent study, over 40 million documented live births were examined by the Centers for Disease Control and Prevention and the National Center for Health Statistics database between 2007 and 2016 in the United States[13]. The study investigated the impact of advanced paternal age on maternal and perinatal outcomes and found a higher paternal age was associated with an increased risk of premature birth, low birth weight, and low Apgar score. Although as of the time of writing clear evidence is not available that sperm selection technologies provide dramatic improvement in improving pregnancy rates, a common theme in such studies has been reduction in miscarriage rates.

How will sperm be prepared and selected in the future? The most promising methodology will likely involve selection via a microfluidic platform for IVF/ICSI cases[14]. These platforms have already entered into a testing phase in many IVF laboratories[15]. For example, in the early 2000s, Takayama and Smith used two parallel laminar flow channels where nonmotile spermatozoa and debris would flow along their initial streamlines and exit one outlet, whereas motile spermatozoa had an opportunity to swim into a parallel stream and exit a separate outlet. They found that both motility (98%) and morphology (22%) improved significantly[16].

Relying solely on the motility characteristics and size to sort sperm by microfluidics will most likely be surpassed by further innovations to these systems. Already, we have seen the addition of chemoattractants to further help separate sperm in a microfluidics platform[17,18]. Addition of cumulus cells in a microfluidic chamber, to act as the chemoattractant, helped increase the percentage of motile sperms from 58.5% to 82.6% [18]. A further addition will definitely be the integration of optics into the selection process[19]. One of the most interesting applications for integrating microfluidics and optics may be the use of Raman spectroscopy, which has already been shown to distinguish sperm with improved nuclear integrity[20].

The IVF Laboratory Processes

It is envisaged that several aspects of clinical embryology over the coming decades, including ICSI, embryo culture, and cryopreservation, have the potential to become automated. Such advances may be achieved through microrobotics and microfluidic systems, which are already being adapted into many processes of IVF (Figure 5.2).

Egg Collection and Processing

The first step in an IVF procedure is to collect oocytes. There have been no automated and continuous processing systems that can reduce the dependence on well-trained embryologists to obtain ICSI-ready oocytes from patients. Recently, however, using mouse models, a microfluidic device to denude oocytes from the surrounding cumulus-corona cell mass was reported[21]. Oocytes that were denuded by the device showed comparable fertilization and developmental competence compared with mechanical

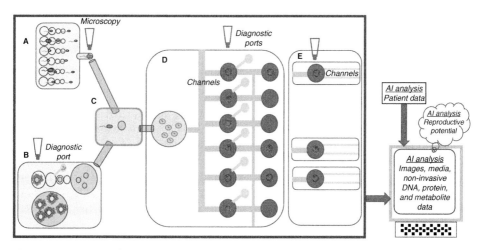

Figure 5.2 Integration of microfluidic systems for (A) sperm selection, (B) egg collection, (C) insemination/ICSI, (D) embryo culture, and (E) cryopreservation. All stages are monitored by noninvasive microscopy involving time-lapse, image recognition, fluorescence-lifetime imaging microscopy (FLIM), and spectroscopy, while diagnostic ports are able to collect DNA, protein, and metabolites for analysis. Computer-controlled channels will allow input and output of fluids to allow gamete/embryo movement and to individualize culture conditions related to developmental stage. Channels will also allow control of cryopreservation to maximize vitrification and warming. All gamete and embryo data will be integrated with individual patient data to allow artificial intelligence (AI) to construct a reproductive health assessment of each embryo.

pipetting. The device allows access to denuded oocytes that would be ready for either ICSI or vitrification.

ICSI and Routine Insemination

The advent of ICSI[22] revolutionized the treatment of the infertile male. Its adaptation in the IVF laboratory has surpassed its traditionally intended role and it is now applied to nearly 70% of cases worldwide[23]. In many clinics it is used in 100% of cases. The automation of this skill has been attempted by various groups in recent years[24]. In particular, the group of Sun in Toronto has used a robotic system to track sperm and inject them with variable success[25]. None of these systems have been clinically adopted as yet. However, another approach could be via the use of microfluidics.

Although the use of ICSI has been adopted on a more regular basis, the use of microfluidics may allow more improved access of sperm to oocytes in smaller chambers, similar to that seen in the oviduct or fallopian tube. In fact, microfluidics may better mimic oocyte sperm interactions in drastically reduced volumes (mimicking those present in the female tract), allowing for fertilization rates to be achieved with minimal numbers of surrounding spermatozoa. Han and colleagues[26] developed a microwell array used to capture and hold individual oocytes during the flow-through process of oocyte and sperm loading, medium substitution, and debris cleaning. Different micro-well depths were compared by computational modeling and flow washing experiments for their effectiveness in oocyte trapping and debris removal. Fertilization was achieved in the microfluidic devices with similar fertilization rates to controls. The use of shorter exposure and low sperm numbers for insemination has long been argued to improve embryo quality[27] and the use of these systems may translate to improvements in not only process but outcomes.

Embryo Culture

Our ability to culture preimplantation embryos has improved dramatically over the last 40 years. Incubators, culture media, and culture environment have significantly improved and can now facilitate development of the fertilized oocyte to the blastocyst stage in all laboratories[28,29,30]. Although many aspects of embryo culture have improved, the actual hardware we culture embryos in has not changed. Standard culture conditions still call for an embryo to be grown in a petri dish using relatively large media volumes, when compared to embryo size, under oil. The major change in embryo culture in the past 10 years has been in the utilization of time-lapse systems, which has allowed clinics to assess embryos in a continuous temperature and gas phase without environmental perturbations. A number of studies have now shown that the time-lapse systems surpass the older standard incubators[31,32,33] indicating that one benefit may definitely be a nondisturbed environment[34].

One of the unperceived advantages that coincides with time-lapse incubation is the use of specifically designed culture wells that are able to better create microenvironments around the embryo. These wells are characterized by lower incubation volumes per embryo, and by their columnar design in which embryos reside in the base of a small column of medium. These changes to dish design alone have been shown to improve embryo development, compared to that seen in a conventional petri dish in drops of medium under oil[35].

The concept of a nondisturbed environment for culture lends itself well to microfluidic culture systems. Various microfluidic platforms have already been tested in human IVF programs[36]. Some of the original studies reported by Heo and colleagues [37] cultured mouse embryos in a microfluidic system and found that blastocyst development was significantly enhanced in development to the hatching stage and in the average number of cells per blastocyst. Importantly, dynamic microfluidic culture (in which embryos moved) significantly improved embryo implantation and OPRs over static culture to levels approaching that of in utero derived preimplantation embryos[36]. Unfortunately, although many systems have been developed that allow microfluidic embryo culture to be performed, their adaptation has yet to be realized. However, this could change in the future as the microfluidic platforms also allow two major adjunct improvements to embryo culture. Firstly, they allow the manipulation of the media so that it can better suit the dynamic nature of preimplantation embryo development[38]. The adoption of single-step culture media, although perceived to be equivalent to sequential, does not cater to the embryos' real metabolic needs. Microfluidics will allow these metabolic needs to be synchronized more closely to embryo stages. For example, we envisage a future where embryos are monitored individually and, as they progress in development, they are exposed to changing gradients of nutrients to maximize the physiology of each stage[39]. This could be performed for multiple factors including carbohydrates[40], amino acids[28,41,42], vitamins, growth factors, cytokines[43], and macromolecules. More importantly, interactive culture systems could be developed whereby embryo culture may finally be able to mimic that of an in vivo environment. In a recent study by Ferraz and colleagues[44], bovine embryos were cultured in a microfluidic chamber in addition to oviductal feeder cells. The authors concluded that cultured embryos were able to show in vivo characteristics as culture using "oviduct-on-a-chip". This culture system yielded 50% of zygotes with no discernible difference in gene expression pattern when compared to in vivo zygotes. They postulated that their results highlight the importance of a more in vivo like environment when studying pathways related to normal fertilization and zygote formation in vitro and suggested that future studies should focus on the relevance of this improved environment for further (epi)genetic reprogramming events in developing embryos.

A second benefit of microfluidic platforms is the ability to perform in line diagnostics of embryos as they are growing. This concept was proven by Urbanski and colleagues [45], who showed that a microfluidic device could be employed in which media samples are loaded or integrated into microfluidic culture systems for in-line, real-time metabolic evaluation. As a proof of principle, metabolic activities of single murine embryos were evaluated using this device. Interestingly, they also adapted the use of a standard epifluorescent microscope and a charge-coupled device camera to their system, which opens up further possibilities of incorporating other diagnostic technologies covered later in this chapter.

Embryo Cryopreservation

Since the first report of a frozen IVF pregnancy in 1983 by Trounson and Mohr[46], embryo cryopreservation has become a major part of any IVF cycle. Although embryo freezing was able to provide limited successes, the advent of vitrification has revolutionized freezing of eggs and embryos to the extent that frozen embryo transfers are now surpassing fresh transfers as an option for ET[47,48]. In the future it is plausible that the current benefits seen in the transfer of vitrified embryos will translate to all cycles being completed by a frozen ET. In addition, change in clinical practice may provide a better luteal support and improve live birth outcomes[49].

The challenges to improving freezing protocols are related to both time and outcome efficiency. Automated vitrification systems are already under development, which are aimed at improving laboratory efficiency[50,51]. A further improvement will be the ability to provide greater control over the cryopreservation process. For example, the group of Sun[52] has described a digital microfluidic device that automates sample preparation for mammalian embryo vitrification. The automated operation allowed gametes or embryos to pass through a cryoprotectant concentration gradient, which is distinct from current practice where they are passed through several steps of solutions. This in itself may improve outcomes. Further refinements may also involve the ability to visually monitor individual eggs or embryos during the cryopreservation process and adjust the addition of cryoprotectants to each egg or embryo, which may be of greatest significance in a population of oocytes from older patients. In the future, therefore, we may provide "personalized egg or embryo freezing" through a combination of optical and microfluidic techniques.

Egg and Embryo Analysis

The development of precise methods for assessing oocyte and embryo quality has long remained a critical goal in ART. Forty years after the first IVF procedures were performed, morphological assessment remains the primary method of evaluation, despite its well-known limitations[53]. Morphological features per se, however, have no clear connection to the underlying biochemical factors that are essential for viability, such as metabolic function and genetic integrity[54]. However, using time lapse to quantitate the timing of key events, such as initiation of cavitation to full blastocoel expansion, could well be linked to metabolic activity over a defined period[53]. Current technology for embryo assessment is largely based on biopsy of the trophectoderm followed by genetic analysis. This, however, has raised a number of concerns not only because the procedure is invasive and requires removal of cells from the embryo, but also because it is only representative of part of the embryo. We consider that in future these tests will be superseded by noninvasive testing, which will give a more holistic evaluation of the entire embryo and will provide information about genetic, metabolic, and transcriptional activity, thereby not only reflecting the ploidy and viability of the embryo but providing important information regarding the health of the embryo itself[3].

Metabolic

The metabolic state of an embryo is not only predictive of viability (defined as the ability to implant) but is also reflective of the actual health of the embryo (as defined by the development of the resultant fetus). To date, assessment of metabolic function has relied heavily on specialized miniaturized procedures, available to only a few laboratories worldwide. Noninvasive embryo assessment of the embryo's metabolic state can now be performed indirectly through a number of novel imaging platforms, which can obtain information about the metabolic functions of the embryo. Raman spectroscopy, Fourier transform infrared spectroscopy, or FLIM and hyperspectral analysis can all be used to provide additional spectroscopic data on embryos, and they thus have the potential to produce superior clinical tools for embryo assessment[55,56]. One methodology that has recently provided interesting data on mouse eggs and embryos is FLIM[57]. Interestingly, experiments on mouse oocytes have shown that FLIM parameters exhibit strong differentiation between old versus young oocytes. FLIM could potentially be used as a noninvasive tool to assess mitochondrial function in oocytes and can also discriminate between oocytes that have had their mitochondria genetically manipulated. Other types of microscopic analysis are also being examined in the realm of embryology. Hyperspectral analysis investigates overall autofluorescent signatures and their cellular distribution. Like FLIM, this technique has also been shown in other cell systems to provide insights into cellular processes, including embryos. Recently, this type of analysis was shown for the first time to extract noninvasively, biologically relevant, and quantitative information from cells and tissues. It was able to identify and document autofluorescence by multispectral imaging whereby a spectrum is taken at each pixel in the image, generating about a million such spectra from cellular areas with varying molecular composition[57]. Individual cells are segmented out and their images processed to generate multiple, mathematically defined cellular features. The endogenous cell fluorophores examined included nicotinamide adenine dinucleotide, nicotinamide adenine dinucleotide phosphate, flavin adenine dinucleotide, flavin mononucleotide, N-retinylidene-N-retinylethanolamine, cytochrome C, and proteins including abundant species like collagen and elastin. The ability of these novel optical methods may be integrated in egg and embryo assessment in the future laboratory. It is plausible that such systems will be combined with microfluidic platforms to provide real-time embryo analysis.

Genetic
Noninvasive/Semi-Invasive PGT

At the time of writing, the most reliable embryo analysis technology is PGT-A using trophectodermal biopsies. This technology consistently provides greater than 50% live birth rates when a euploid embryo is found for transfer (see Chapter 2). Unfortunately, the technique requires significant laboratory resources, including the actual trophectoderm biopsy itself and the addition of cryopreservation of all blastocysts prior to analysis. Recently, however, the advent of noninvasive PGT-A may circumvent much of the need for biopsying embryos. Promising noninvasive methods to genetically analyze the embryo include blastocoelic fluid[58] and/or media assessment[59,] and the use of advanced microscopy techniques[60,61]. In several years' time, the need to biopsy an embryo will most likely be unnecessary.

AI

Through the introduction of time-lapse microscopy, we are now in the unique position of collecting more data than a clinical embryology laboratory can utilize. With embryos being imaged every 10 minutes, during a 4- to 5-day culture period, over 700 pictures (each with several focal planes) are amassed, therefore taking the total number of images available for consideration into the thousands (and to think we used to look at embryos once each day, giving a total of 5 or so images on which to make our decisions!). With the ability to annotate embryo development, and the application of algorithms to model the significance of discrete events, we can now utilize the potential of time-lapse to a greater extent than first imagined[54,62,63]. However, even the most sophisticated algorithms to date use only a small percent of the available information. AI is a means to maximize the potential of time-lapse microscopy in clinical IVF[64]. Rather than taking a sample of images into consideration, AI can utilize every image at every focal plane, in order to learn what time-dependent features are associated with successful transfer outcome, such as fetal heart rate[65]. Furthermore, AI will be of value in integrating the growing amount of clinical data collected per embryo, allowing patient parameters to also be combined into decision-making with the images acquired throughout development.

A final benefit of AI in combination with microfluidics will be added safety for tracking patients' gametes and embryos, allowing all the data to be assimilated into electronic medical records, which would include witnessing systems. This will allow patients' gametes and embryos to be tracked more efficiently with the ultimate aim of eliminating any errors in the laboratory[66].

Non-IVF Related Technologies in the IVF Laboratory

The IVF laboratory of the future may not only process eggs and embryos. It may be critical in creating gametes from stem cells. We have already seen numerous advances in creating gametes from stem cells and in animals, in which researchers have obtained live offspring[67–70]. Furthermore, in vitro maturation (IVM) may play a greater role in the treatment of infertility. This may be via stem cells or in the harvesting of immature follicles. Extensive research in this area[71] is now reawakening the possibility of using IVM in clinical IVF, beyond the treatment of polycystic ovarian syndrome (PCOS) cases [72]. Finally, the laboratory of the future may also be implicated in treatment of inheritable genetic diseases. Technologies such as clustered regularly interspaced short palindromic repeats may be implemented in modifying embryos for patients[68] and embryo selection may also involve calculating polygenic risk[73]. In implementing such technologies, the challenging ethical decisions centered on an IVF laboratory will remain, just as they were prevalent when Bob Edwards reported the first IVF baby.

Conclusion

The initial laboratory conditions responsible for the creation of Louise Brown have changed significantly over the intervening decades. We predict that more changes will be forthcoming through innovation in automation, microrobotics, and microfluidics, all combined with AI. Hence, the laboratory of tomorrow is more likely to be an integral component in "personalized medicine" to better diagnose and treat couples. Clinical profiles will be fundamental to choosing how a patient's gametes and embryos are monitored individually as they progress in development. Culture and selection could be performed in a microfluidic device allowing greater efficiency, safety, and overall efficacy in the laboratory. Gamete and embryo data created, via imaging and media sampling for metabolites and DNA, will be integrated into algorithms that could also incorporate the couple's own clinical profile. This will allow a truly personalized approach in handling the gametes and embryos of each patient in the laboratory. Importantly, such an approach will enable the laboratory to maximize each couple's chance of achieving a healthy singleton live birth. It should also provide a rapid and meaningful diagnosis in the advent of a failed cycle, thereby facilitating the patient to be treated efficiently in future treatment cycles, or even to provide closure in the event of extremely poor prognosis. Ultimately, however, the approaches considered will improve laboratory efficiencies and reduce time to pregnancy.

References

1. Menkin MF, Rock J In Vitro Fertilization and Cleavage of Human Ovarian Eggs. *Am J Obstet Gynecol.* 1948.

2. Rock J, MM. In Vitro Fertilization and Cleavage of Human Ovarian Eggs. *Science (80-).* 1944; 100(**2588**): 105–7.

3. Ferrick L, Lee YSL, Gardner DK. Reducing Time to Pregnancy and Facilitating the Birth of Healthy Children through Functional Analysis of Embryo Physiology. *Biol Reprod.* 2019.

4. Sati L, Bennett D, Janes M, Huszar G. Next Day Determination of Ejaculatory Sperm Motility After Overnight Shipment of Semen to Remote Locations. *J Assist Reprod Genet.* 2015; 32(**1**): 117–25.

5. Kanakasabapathy MK, Sadasivam M, Singh A, Preston C, Thirumalaraju P, Venkataraman M, et al. An Automated Smartphone-Based Diagnostic Assay for Point-of-Care Semen Analysis. *Sci Transl Med.* 2017; 9(**382**).

6. Agarwal et al. Male Oxidative Stress Infertility (MOSI): Proposed Terminology and Clinical Practice Guidelines for Management of Idiopathic Male Infertility. *World J Men's Health.* 2019; 37(**3**): 296–312.

7. Jenkins TG, Aston KI, James ER, Carrell DT. Sperm Epigenetics in the Study of Male Fertility, Offspring Health, and Potential Clinical Applications. *Syst Biol Reprod Med.* 2017; 63(**2**): 69–76.

8. Jodar M, Sendler E, Moskovtsev SI, Librach CL, Goodrich R, Swanson S, et al. Absence of Sperm RNA Elements Correlates with Idiopathic Male Infertility. *Sci Transl Med.* 2015; 7(**295**).

9. Jodar M, Sendler E, Krawetz SA. The Protein and Transcript Profiles of Human Semen. *Cell Tissue Res.* 2016; 363(**1**): 85–96.

10. Jodar M, Selvaraju S, Sendler E, Diamond MP, Krawetz SA. The Presence, Role and Clinical Use of Spermatozoal RNAs. *Hum Reprod Update.* 2013; 19(**6**): 604–24.

11. Jenkins TG, Aston KI, Pflueger C, Cairns BR, Carrell DT. Age-Associated Sperm DNA Methylation Alterations: Possible Implications in Offspring Disease Susceptibility. *PLoS Genet.* 2014; 10(**7**): e1004458.

12. Carrell DT, Aston KI, Oliva R, Emery BR, De Jonge CJ. The "Omics" of Human Male Infertility: Integrating Big Data in a Systems Biology Approach. *Cell Tissue Res.* 2016.

13. Khandwala YS, Zhang CA, Lu Y, Eisenberg ML. The Age of Fathers in the USA Is Rising: An Analysis of 168 867 480 Births from 1972 to 2015. *Hum Reprod.* 2017; 32(**10**): 2110–16.

14. Vaughan DA, Sakkas D. Sperm Selection Methods in the 21st Century. *Biol Reprod.*

15. de Wagenaar B, Berendsen JTW, Bomer JG, Olthuis W, van den Berg A, Segerink LI. Microfluidic Single Sperm Entrapment and Analysis. *Lab Chip.* 2015; 15(**5**): 1294–301.

16. Smith GD, Takayama S. Application of Microfluidic Technologies to Human Assisted Reproduction. *Mol Hum Reprod.* 2017; gaw076.

17. Bhagwat S, Sontakke S, KD, Parte P, Jadhav S. Chemotactic Behavior of Spermatozoa Captured Using a Microfluidic Chip. *Biomicrofluidics.* 2018; 12(**2**): 024112.

18. Ko Y-J, Maeng J-H, Hwang SY, Ahn Y. Design, Fabrication, and Testing of a Microfluidic Device for Thermotaxis and Chemotaxis Assays of Sperm. *SLAS Technol.* 2018; 23(**6**): 507–15.

19. Eravuchira PJ, Mirsky SK, Barnea I, Levi M, Balberg M, Shaked NT. Individual Sperm Selection by Microfluidics Integrated with Interferometric Phase Microscopy. *Methods.* 2018; 136: 152–9.

20. Amaral S, Da Costa R, Wübbeling F, Redmann K, Schlatt S. Raman Micro-Spectroscopy Analysis of Different

Sperm Regions: A Species Comparison. *MHR Basic Sci Reprod Med*. 2018;24 (**4**): 185–202.

21. Weng L, Lee GY, Liu J, Kapur R, Toth TL, Toner M. On-Chip Oocyte Denudation from Cumulus–Oocyte Complexes for Assisted Reproductive Therapy. *Lab Chip*. 2018; 18(**24**): 3892–902.

22. Palermo G, Joris H, Devroey P, Van Steirteghem AC. Pregnancies After Intracytoplasmic Injection of Single Spermatozoon into an Oocyte. *Lancet*. 1992; 340(**8810**): 17–18.

23. Adamson GD, de Mouzon J, Chambers GM, Zegers-Hochschild F, Mansour R, Ishihara O, et al. International Committee for Monitoring Assisted Reproductive Technology: World Report on Assisted Reproductive Technology. *Fertil Steril*. 2011; 110(**6**): 1067–80.

24. Zhang Z, Dai C, Huang JY, Wang X, Liu J, Ru C, et al. Robotic Immobilization of Motile Sperm for Clinical Intracytoplasmic Sperm Injection. *IEEE Trans Biomed Eng*. 2018.

25. Lu Z, Zhang X, Leung C, Esfandiari N, Casper RF, Sun Y. Robotic ICSI (Intracytoplasmic Sperm Injection). *IEEE Trans Biomed Eng* 2011.

26. Han C, Zhang Q, Ma R, Xie L, Qiu T, Wang L, et al. Integration of Single Oocyte Trapping, in Vitro Fertilization and Embryo Culture in a Microwell-Structured Microfluidic Device. *Lab Chip*. 2010.

27. Kattera S, Chen C. Short Coincubation of Gametes in in Vitro Fertilization Improves Implantation and Pregnancy Rates: A Prospective, Randomized, Controlled Study. *Fertil Steril*. 2003; 80(**4**): 1017–21.

28. Bavister BD. Culture of Preimplantation Embryos: Facts and Artifacts. *Hum Reprod Update*. 1995; 1(**2**): 91–148.

29. Gardner DK, Lane M. Culture of viable mammalian embryos. In: Cibelli J, Lanza R, Campbell K, West M (eds.), Principles of Cloning. San Diego: Academic Press. 2014; 63–84.

30. Gardner DK, Lane M. Culture systems for the human embryo. In: Gardner DK, Weissman A, Howles C, Shoham Z (eds.) Textbook of Assisted Reproductive Techniques. Informa Healthcare. 2018; 200–24.

31. Pribenszky C, Nilselid A-M, Montag M. Time-Lapse Culture with Morphokinetic Embryo Selection Improves Pregnancy and Live Birth Chances and Reduces Early Pregnancy Loss: A Meta-Analysis. *Reprod Biomed Online*. 2017; 35(**5**): 511–20.

32. Paulson RJ, Reichman DE, Zaninovic N, Goodman LR, Racowsky C. Time-Lapse Imaging: Clearly Useful to Both Laboratory Personnel and Patient Outcomes Versus Just Because We Can Doesn't Mean We Should. *Fertil Steril*. 2018; 109(**4**): 584–91.

33. Armstrong S, Bhide P, Jordan V, Pacey A, Farquhar C. Time-Lapse Systems for Embryo Incubation and Assessment in Assisted Reproduction. *Cochrane database Syst Rev*. 2018; 5:CD011320.

34. Wale PL, Gardner DK. The Effects of Chemical and Physical Factors on Mammalian Embryo Culture and Their Importance for the Practice of Assisted Human Reproduction. *Hum Reprod Update*. 2016; 22(**1**): 2–22.

35. Gardner DK, Kelley RL. Impact of the IVF Laboratory Environment on Human Preimplantation Embryo Phenotype. *J Dev Orig Health Dis*. 2017; 8(**4**): 418–35.

36. Bormann C, Cabrera L, Heo YS, Takayama S, Smith G. Dynamic Microfluidic Embryo Culture Enhances Blastocyst Development of Murine and Bovine Embryos. *Biol Reprod*. 2017.

37. Heo YS, Cabrera LM, Bormann CL, Shah CT, Takayama S, Smith GD. Dynamic Microfunnel Culture Enhances Mouse Embryo Development and Pregnancy Rates. *Hum Reprod*. 2010.

38. Gardner DK, Pool TB, Lane M. Embryo Nutrition and Energy Metabolism and Its Relationship to Embryo Growth, Differentiation, and Viability. *Semin Reprod Med*. 2000.

39. Gardner DK. Mammalian Embryo Culture in the Absence of Serum or Somatic Cell Support. *Cell Biol Int.*; 18 (**12**): 1163–79.

40. Gardner DK, Sakkas D. Mouse Embryo Cleavage, Metabolism and Viability: Role of Medium Composition. *Hum Reprod.* 1993; 8(**2**).

41. Steeves TE, Gardner DK. Temporal and Differential Effects of Amino Acids on Bovine Embryo Development in Culture. *Biol Reprod.* 1999; 61(**3**): 731–40.

42. Lane M, Gardner DK. Differential Regulation of Mouse Embryo Development and Viability by Amino Acids. *J Reprod Fertil.* 1997; 109(**1**): 153–64.

43. Thouas GA, Dominguez F, Green MP, Vilella F, Simon C, Gardner DK. Soluble Ligands and Their Receptors in Human Embryo Development and Implantation. *Endocrine Rev.* 2015; 36(**1**): 92–130.

44. Ferraz MAMM, Rho HS, Hemerich D, Henning HHW, van Tol HTA, Hölker M, et al. An Oviduct-on-a-Chip Provides an Enhanced in Vitro Environment for Zygote Genome Reprogramming. *Nat Commun.* 2018.

45. Urbanski JP, Johnson MT, Craig DD, Potter DL, Gardner DK, Thorsen T. Noninvasive Metabolic Profiling Using Microfluidics for Analysis of Single Preimplantation Embryos. *Anal Chem.* 2008; 80(**17**): 6500–7.

46. Trounson A, Mohr L. Human Pregnancy Following Cryopreservation, Thawing and Transfer of an Eight-Cell Embryo. *Nature.* 1983.

47. Lane M, Schoolcraft WB, Gardner DK. Vitrification of Mouse and Human Blastocysts Using a Novel Cryoloop Container-less Technique. *Fertil Steril.* 1999; 72(**6**): 1073–8.

48. Rienzi L, Gracia C, Maggiulli R, LaBarbera AR, Kaser DJ, Ubaldi FM, et al. Oocyte, Embryo and Blastocyst Cryopreservation in ART: Systematic Review and Meta-Analysis Comparing Slow-Freezing Versus Vitrification to Produce Evidence for the Development of Global Guidance. *Hum Reprod Update.* 2016.

49. von Versen-Höynck F, Schaub AM, Chi Y-Y, Chiu K-H, Liu J, Lingis M, et al. Increased Preeclampsia Risk and Reduced Aortic Compliance With in Vitro Fertilization Cycles in the Absence of a Corpus Luteum. *Hypertens.* 1979; 73(**3**): 640–9.

50. Roy TK, Brandi S, Peura TT. Chapter 20 Gavi-Automated Vitrification Instrument. *Methods Mol Biol.* 2017; 1568: 261–77.

51. Arav A, Natan Y, Kalo D, Komsky-Elbaz A, Roth Z, Levi-Setti PE, et al. A New, Simple, Automatic Vitrification Device: Preliminary Results with Murine and Bovine Oocytes and Embryos. *J Assist Reprod Genet.* 2018; 35(**7**): 1161–8.

52. Pyne DG, Liu J, Abdelgawad M, Sun Y. Digital Microfluidic Processing of Mammalian Embryos for Vitrification. *PLoS One.* 2014; 9(**9**): e108128.

53. Gardner DK, Balaban B. Assessment of Human Embryo Development Using Morphological Criteria in an Era of Time-Lapse, Algorithms and "OMICS": Is Looking Good Still Important? *Mol Hum Reprod.* 2016; 22(**10**): 704–18.

54. Gardner DK, Meseguer M, Rubio C, Treff NR. Diagnosis of Human Preimplantation Embryo Viability. *Hum Reprod Update.* 2015; 21(**6**): 727–47.

55. Sanchez T, Seidler EA, Gardner DK, Needleman D, Sakkas D. Will Noninvasive Methods Surpass Invasive for Assessing Gametes and Embryos? *Fertil Steril.* 2017; 108(**5**): 730–7.

56. Gardner DK, Reineck P, Gibson BC, Thompson J. Microfluidics and Microanalytics to Facilitate Quantitative Assessment of Human Embryo Physiology. In: Agarwal A, Varghese A, Nagy ZP (eds.) Practical Manual of In Vitro Fertilization: Advanced Methods and Novel Devices. New Jersey: Humana Press. 2019.

57. Sanchez T, Wang T, Pedro MV, Zhang M, Esencan E, Sakkas D, et al. Metabolic Imaging with the Use of Fluorescence

Lifetime Imaging Microscopy (FLIM) Accurately Detects Mitochondrial Dysfunction in Mouse Oocytes. *Fertil Steril*. 2018; 110(**7**): 1387–97.

58. Capalbo A, Romanelli V, Patassini C, Poli M, Girardi L, Giancani A, et al. Diagnostic Efficacy of Blastocoel Fluid and Spent Media as Sources of DNA for Preimplantation Genetic Testing in Standard Clinical Conditions. *Fertil Steril*. 2018; 110(**5**): 870–9.e5

59. Xu J, Fang R, Chen L, Chen D, Xiao J-P, Yang W, et al. Noninvasive Chromosome Screening of Human Embryos by Genome Sequencing of Embryo Culture Medium for in Vitro Fertilization. *Proc Natl Acad Sci USA*. 2016; 113(**42**): 11907–12.

60. Sutton-McDowall ML, Gosnell M, Anwer AG, White M, Purdey M, Abell AD, et al. Hyperspectral Microscopy Can Detect Metabolic Heterogeneity Within Bovine Post-Compaction Embryos Incubated under Two Oxygen Concentrations (7% Versus 20%). *Hum Reprod*. 2017; 32(**10**): 2016–25.

61. Sanchez T, Wang T, Pedro MV, Zhang M, Esencan E, Sakkas D, et al. Metabolic Imaging with the Use of Fluorescence Lifetime Imaging Microscopy (FLIM) Accurately Detects Mitochondrial Dysfunction in Mouse Oocytes. *Fertil Steril*. 2018; 110(**7**).

62. Liu Y, Chapple V, Feenan K, Roberts P, Matson P. Time-Lapse Deselection Model for Human Day 3 in Vitro Fertilization Embryos: The Combination of Qualitative and Quantitative Measures of Embryo Growth. *Fertil Steril*. 2016; 105(**3**): 656–62.e1.

63. Petersen BM, Boel M, Montag M, Gardner DK. Development of a Generally Applicable Morphokinetic Algorithm Capable of Predicting the Implantation Potential of Embryos Transferred on Day 3. *Hum Reprod*. 2016; 31(**10**).

64. Khosravi P, Kazemi E, Zhan Q, Malmsten JE, Toschi M, Zisimopoulos P, et al. Deep Learning Enables Robust Assessment and Selection of Human Blastocysts After in Vitro Fertilization. *Nat Digit Med*. 2019; 2.

65. Tran A, Cooke S, Illingworth PJ, Gardner DK. A Study of the Diagnostic Accuracy of Deep Learning, a Novel Approach for Predicting the Fetal Heart Implantation Rate Following Time-Lapse Incubation. *Hum Reprod*. 2019; in press.

66. Sakkas D, Brent Barrett C, Alper MM. Types and Frequency of Non-Conformances in an IVF Laboratory. *Hum Reprod*. 2018; 33(**12**).

67. Nagamatsu G, Hayashi K. Stem Cells, in Vitro Gametogenesis and Male Fertility. *Reproduction*. 2017; 154(**6**): F79–91.

68. Ma H, Marti-Gutierrez N, Park S-W, Wu J, Lee Y, Suzuki K, et al. Correction of a Pathogenic Gene Mutation in Human Embryos. *Nature*. 2017; 548(**7668**): 413–19.

69. Hayashi K, Ogushi S, Kurimoto K, Shimamoto S, Ohta H, Saitou M. Offspring from Oocytes Derived from in Vitro Primordial Germ Cell-like Cells in Mice. *Science (80-)*. 2012; 338(**6109**): 971–5.

70. Hayashi K, Saitou M. Generation of Eggs from Mouse Embryonic Stem Cells and Induced Pluripotent Stem Cells. *Nat Protoc*. 2013; 8(**8**): 1513–24.

71. Richani D, Constance K, Lien S, Agapiou D, Stocker WA, Hedger MP, et al. Cumulin and FSH Cooperate to Regulate Inhibin B and Activin B Production by Human Granulosa-Lutein Cells In Vitro. *Endocrinology*. 2019; 160(**4**): 853–62.

72. Vuong LN, Ho VNA, Ho TM, Dang VQ, Phung TH, Giang NH, et al. Effectiveness and Safety of in Vitro Maturation of Oocytes Versus in Vitro Fertilisation in Women with High Antral Follicle Count: Study Protocol for a Randomised Controlled Trial. 2018; 8(**12**): e023413.

73. Treff NR, Zimmerman R, Bechor E, Hsu J, Rana B, Jensen J, et al. Validation of Concurrent Preimplantation Genetic Testing for Polygenic and Monogenic Disorders, Structural Rearrangements, and Whole and Segmental Chromosome Aneuploidy with a Single Universal Platform. *Eur J Med Genet*. 2019.

6

Integrative Care

Sarah R Holley and Lauri A Pasch

> There are no psychosocial problems without biological features, and there are no biomedical problems without psychosocial features.

McDaniel, Doherty, and Hepworth, 2015

Couples (or individuals) present for fertility treatment because they are unable to conceive a viable pregnancy on their own. From a purely medical model perspective, the goal is fairly straightforward: to achieve a pregnancy in patients who would otherwise not have been able to do so, using a menu of reproductive technology options. This medical model approach may not be the best way to comprehensively care for patients, however. The approach tends to ignore social and behavioral factors that may impact outcomes, assumes that patients will remain in care until the anticipated pregnancy is achieved (or is determined to be no longer possible by the physician), and places relatively greater emphasis on achievement of pregnancy than on healthy outcomes for mother and child. Some fertility treatment centers have been shifting toward a patient-centered care model that provides an integrated set of services including medical, psychosocial, behavioral, dietary, and alternative interventions. This integrative care approach encourages treatment providers to look more holistically at the patient or couple and deliver care that meets a spectrum of needs.

The goal of this chapter is to examine the delivery of integrative care within a reproductive endocrinology and infertility (REI) clinic setting. The chapter will first examine the nature of integrative care, and why this type of approach may be particularly applicable to fertility treatment patients. It will then review some of the possible components that may be included in an integrative care system, and explore examples of different approaches clinics can take to provide integrated services. We will examine additional considerations related to certain treatment groups, and conclude with a call for providers to consider ways they can use integrative models of care in order to best serve their patients' family-building goals.

What is Integrative Care and Why is it Useful?

In the United States, the medical system has in many ways taken a reductionist approach that views medical problems as a set of symptoms that must be fixed. Practitioners become specialists who focus on addressing their singular piece of the problem. The health insurance industry reinforces this system – a specific problem within a specific organ system must be identified, then a specific tool applied. Anything outside this limited system falls outside the purview of treatment or insurance coverage. The result is often fragmented, impersonal, and costly care[1].

Calls to address this medical model issue have been around for some time. In 1977, George Engel published a seminal article in *Science* calling for a new approach. He observed that the "concentration on the biomedical and exclusion of the psychosocial distorts perspectives and even interferes with patient care[2]". Engel proposed a new biopsychosocial model that would take into account the patient's thoughts, feelings, and behaviors related to illness and care, as well as the larger social and cultural context in which the care was occurring.

In the decades since, the drumbeat to provide patient care that cuts across disciplines and more effectively addresses the spectrum of patient needs has only increased. The type of biopsychosocial approach that Engel proposed has come to be referred to as *integrative care*. As applied to medical care, the integrative care model is defined as the delivery of treatment in a way that "reaffirms the importance of the relationship between practitioner and patient, focuses on the whole person, is informed by evidence, and makes use of all appropriate therapeutic and lifestyle approaches, healthcare professionals and disciplines to achieve optimal health and healing[3]". Integrative care typically has medical, psychological, and a mixture of other services that are collectively incorporated within a patient's treatment plan[4]. As will be explored below, integrative care is related to, but conceptually different from, collaborative care. Collaborative care is characterized by a "multidisciplinary approach," where each provider completes their task in an additive way; integrative care moves toward an "interdisciplinary approach" wherein members of the healthcare team work together with a set of shared goals[5].

Infertility in particular warrants such an integrative, biopsychosocial approach to care. For example, take the case of a heterosexual couple presenting for treatment. Both members of the couple are in their early thirties. They have been trying to get pregnant via intercourse for a year now. They started casually, but then attempts were increasingly timed around ovulation. They cannot understand why they are not having success when everyone around them seems to be getting pregnant with little to no effort. The woman consults with her gynecologist, who refers her to an REI clinic. There, they undergo a number of medical tests, including sperm count, follicle count, genetic screening, blood tests, and hormone levels. They both wonder if there is a more natural approach that could help them. The doctor recommends a protocol, and the couple moves forward. They must accept that thousands of dollars will be spent toward a treatment with a limited chance of success. They must tolerate the waiting, the lack of control, and the fear of what it means if treatment does not work. Decisions will need to be made, costs and benefits weighed, priorities identified. The wife, who is overweight, wonders, do I need to lose weight? The husband wonders, are we failing because we are so stressed out? They are sad, they are scared, and they desperately want to know what they can do to improve their odds of success.

There is nothing unique about the case described above – that this is typical highlights the myriad challenges that fertility treatment patients (and their providers) face. Other cases may bring up even more questions for the couple . . . do donor gametes need to be used? Where do these come from? Do we tell the child? And if so, how? Additional challenges may be layered on top: physical health concerns, mental health concerns, financial concerns, legal concerns, relationship conflict, lack of family or social support, and so on. No single provider can address all these needs. Thus, it is important to remember that fertility treatment does not happen in a medical vacuum – it is a process that occurs within an evolving ecosystem of providers. The integrative care model aims to deliver the kind of ongoing, interdisciplinary support needed to help patients effectively navigate the biological, psychological, and socioemotional challenges inherent in the treatment process.

Components of Integrative Care

Clinics providing REI services will already have the necessary personnel in place related to the medical care of patients (e.g., physicians, nurses, lab technicians, embryologists, genetic screening). This section will look at specific additional services that clinics can implement when providing care from an integrative framework, which would provide psychosocial benefit to patients as they pursue their family-building goals.

Mental Health Services

Although fertility treatment allows couples to achieve pregnancy who otherwise would not have been able to, each cycle of treatment is more likely to fail than to succeed. As such, fertility treatment is very stressful and is associated with extremely high rates of psychological distress for both partners[6,7]. Psychological distress not only has obvious adverse effects on the well-being of the individual and the couple's relationship, it also reduces the chance of treatment success because it often leads patients to terminate treatment before reaching the ultimate goal of becoming parents[8,9]. Furthermore, working with these highly anxious and depressed patients places significant strain on fertility treatment staff, leading to burnout, lower productivity, and attrition, which are all very costly for clinic functioning[8]. Therefore, integrating mental healthcare providers (MHPs) into fertility treatment serves a number of crucial functions.

The typical role of the MHP includes psychological assessment, psychoeducational support, and counseling of individuals and couples[10]. Counseling goals often include improving ways to cope, making decisions about treatment, or addressing issues between partners. It may also be about dealing with difficult emotions elicited by the diagnosis or treatment, including sadness, guilt, shame, blame, and fear. Other times, treatment may focus on accepting difficult situations and on processing feelings of grief and loss. MHPs can also provide end-of-treatment counseling when treatment is not successful[11]. Cognitive behavioral therapy (CBT)-based interventions in particular have been found to be efficacious in reducing distress[12].

The MHP can also function as an interpreter for the healthcare system. For example, when patients receive difficult or complicated medical information, they often only retain pieces of it or may misperceive what is being said. When care is integrated, the MHP will be in communication with the medical team and will be aware of the patient's diagnosis and treatment plan. In turn, the MHP is well-positioned to offer psychoeducation to the patient or resolve misunderstandings. They can also help information go to the treatment team from the patient, either through direct communication or by helping patients feel empowered to communicate more effectively with the treatment providers[1].

In addition, some (or even much) of the work the MHP does to benefit patients comes via their interactions with other clinic staff members. This can take several forms. For example, in an integrated care model, *all* staff with patient contact (e.g., nurses, doctors, receptionists) are seen as involved in the provision of psychosocial care[13]. The MHP can provide the necessary psychoeducation and training to staff members. Further, just as patients experience a roller coaster of stress and emotions, so too can staff. The MHP can help staff members develop the coping skills needed to avoid burnout or compassion fatigue; this can help to improve communication and reduce negative patient–staff interactions so staff can continue to best serve patients' needs[10]. Finally, more broadly speaking, MHPs are positioned to help clinics assess how they can adjust their service delivery to make treatment less stressful[14]. In this sense, the MHP can move from simply dealing with the stress of treatment to actually making treatment less stressful, thereby improving the experience for patients and staff alike.

Nutritional/Lifestyle Counseling

Maternal diet, weight, and other lifestyle behavioral factors including smoking, substance use, and exposure to toxins undeniably impact the chance of pregnancy as well as maternal and child health outcomes. In fact, obesity has been shown to be so highly associated with IVF success that some providers refuse to treat patients over certain BMI criteria. Recent research argues against this practice based on evidence that lifestyle interventions that delay initiation of IVF are generally ineffective in increasing pregnancy rates. However, it remains clear that weight loss has long-term health benefits for mother and child[15].

The REI doctor working alone is generally ill-equipped to assess and address this multitude of lifestyle and behavioral factors. For example, recent research has shown that fertility physicians acknowledge the importance of screening for eating disorders, but most do not do so and report not feeling confident in their ability to address dietary issues[16]. If lifestyle and dietary issues are not addressed directly by the fertility clinic providers, many patients will go online and discover all sorts of advice about what lifestyle adjustments they should be making in order to conceive. Some people will halt exercise altogether. Others will find tips for the latest fertility-enhancing diet. Unfortunately, certain "interventions" can end up doing more harm than good if they are not based on solid science. For example, a typically active person who ceases all physical activity will notice this takes a major toll on his or her mood and energy level. And some diets can actually do physical harm if a person is losing weight too quickly or not taking in the necessary vitamins and nutrients. Evidence suggests that many patients make behavioral choices that may be detrimental to the goal of healthy pregnancy outcomes[17].

With the goal of promoting healthy pregnancy and optimal maternal and child health outcomes, REI practices should not ignore or refuse patients based on weight or other lifestyle-related behavioral factors, but instead integrate such care into their work. Being able to get detailed, informed answers to their many questions about lifestyle choices can also serve to reduce the stress of fertility patients by providing reassurance, evidence-based guidelines, and supportive interventions as opposed to leaving patients seeking unclear guidance from unreliable sources.

Complementary and Alternative Medicine

Complementary and alternative medicine (CAM) approaches to treating infertility patients have the potential to impact the success of treatment as well as to decrease psychological distress. CAM is broadly defined as "health care approaches that are not typically part of conventional medical care or that may have origins outside of usual Western practice[18]"; these interventions are either used together with medical treatment (complement), or in place of them (alternative). CAM is a very large umbrella: it encompasses natural products, such as vitamins, minerals, and herbal therapy. It also includes "mind/body" practices, such as acupuncture, hypnotherapy, meditation, or relaxation techniques.

It has been estimated that between 30% and 60% of infertility patients use CAM approaches concurrently with their treatment (see review by Boivin and Schmidt[19]). Patients use CAM for a number of reasons. They may feel it is safer, less expensive, or more effective than traditional medical interventions. It may be a first resort, used when difficulty conceiving is first noticed, or a last resort, when confronted with failed fertility treatment cycles or miscarriage. The common denominator is that patients are looking for whatever they can find to move them toward "solving" the fertility problem, and they believe that one or more of these approaches may help.

There is substantial evidence of positive outcomes in the use of CAM approaches. Randomized trials generally support acupuncture as an adjunct to fertility treatment, though results appeared contingent on which control group was considered and various treatment-related factors (e.g., timing of treatment, treatment course)[20]. Another highly promising approach is mind/body interventions, which are shown to be efficacious in reducing distress and may positively impact pregnancy rates[12]. As an example, a recent study evaluated the efficacy of a combined cognitive coping and relaxation intervention (CCRI). Results indicated that the intervention led to improved quality of life and reduced anxiety[21], though it did not appear to improve pregnancy success rates or reduce treatment discontinuation.

CAM interventions appear to be rarely discussed by fertility treatment providers with their patients, presumably because the treatments are generally considered to be at best potentially beneficial and at worst benign. A recent study, however, found that patients who elect for CAM use during treatment may actually experience significantly lower pregnancy rates; this could be because those treatments are most likely to be elected by patients with poor prognosis, but the study controlled for some prognostic factors, suggesting other possible negative mechanisms[19]. Also, when CAM treatments are used outside of the REI clinic, the REI provider is often completely unaware of the nature of the treatment, which could include agents or approaches that are contraindicated (e.g., herbal supplements with endocrine effects). Another risk of participation in CAM treatments is that it may give patients the impression that if they only did one more acupuncture treatment or one more relaxation exercise, they would be more likely to be successful. This can breed inappropriate self-blame if treatment fails[22]. Fertility treatment providers can help patients make informed choices and access safe and appropriate services. Thus, a major benefit of delivering CAM within an integrated setting is that the REI clinic can ensure that patients are receiving only the most evidence-based methods of care that will not work against the clinic's delivery of fertility treatment.

Examples of Different Integrative Approaches

Medical providers can work with other practitioners with varying levels of integration. The level that is right for a given clinic will be determined by a number of factors, including the clinic's infrastructure and the provider's commitment to the integrative model. William Doherty proposed a five-level model for conceptualizing the various configurations of integrative care[23]. These levels are illustrated in Table 6.1.

As highlighted by the MHP example in Table 6.1, the highest level of integrated care is the one most equipped to deal with complex cases with multiple problems and/or providers. Other levels can provide the treatment services needed to achieve a pregnancy, but only at the more integrated levels are the full biopsychosocial spectrum of family-building needs addressed. While a level 5 integrated approach is in theory the gold standard of care, in practice most clinics may not be positioned to achieve this level of integration. Instead, clinics may want to consider what level they are currently at, if that level is working for them (and for their patients), and the relative benefits and costs of trying to move to a higher level of integration.

Collaborative Care

At levels 1 through 3, services are coordinated to varying degrees, but not actually integrated. This would be considered "collaborative care," rather than integrative care. Collaborative care is a partnership of two or more providers who value each other's skills and communicate in a way that enhances the care of patients[1]. Evidence suggests that collaborative care is beneficial for patients. For example, a meta-analysis indicated that interactive communication between primary care physicians and mental health specialists was associated with improved patient outcomes[24]. On-site collaborative care (level 3) has shown additional benefits, including higher physician satisfaction, shorter referral delay, fewer appointments needed, and lower treatment cost[25].

For some clinics, some version of the collaborative model may be what best fits their service model. A relatively small clinic, for example, might not have the financial bandwidth or physical space to add the personnel necessary for an onsite team of integrative providers. Or it may require such a dramatic reconfiguration of practice processes and expansion of expertise that the clinic deems it impractical. Typically, in these cases, clinics practicing with a collaborative model will keep a list of local providers on hand and refer patients out to these services as needed (e.g., for psychological counseling, acupuncture, nutritional counseling, and so on). They may only speak to providers within these referral networks as needed (e.g., in levels 1 and 2, typically driven by specific patient issues), or they may have regular meetings to discuss any current shared patients (e.g., in level 3).

This approach to care, however, comes with a certain set of challenges. When the people with whom a provider is coordinating are not part of their actual practice, collaboration can require a great deal of initiative. As a result, the success (or failure) of the collaborative endeavor will depend on how invested each provider is in the process [4]. If one provider drops the ball in terms of communication, or had different ideas about the direction of the treatment plan, the collaboration will cease to be beneficial. And because there is not within-system accountability, the patient will typically be the one to bear the consequences. In addition, the collaborative model requires patients to follow up on referrals to other providers. This can be a major barrier to care, particularly

Table 6.1 Levels of integration

Level	Description	Example: *REI clinic is treating a patient who is showing symptoms of depression* . . .
1. Minimal collaboration	Medical and mental healthcare and other professionals work in separate facilities, have separate systems, and rarely communicate about cases.	Clinic provides patient with a referral list with the names of several MHPs in the community.
2. Basic collaboration at a distance	Providers have separate systems at separate sites; they engage in periodic communication about shared patients. Providers at each site are viewed as resources and have active referral linkages; communication is driven by specific patient issues.	Clinic refers patient specifically to an MHP in the community with whom they work regularly. When patient begins therapy several weeks later, the MHP contacts the doctor to confirm understanding of patient's medical treatment plan.
3. Basic collaboration on site	Providers have separate systems, but share the same facilities; they engage in regular communication about shared patients. The importance of each other's roles is appreciated, although providers do not share a common language and teams are poorly defined. Physicians have more power and influence over case management decisions than other providers, which can cause tension.	Clinic refers patient to an MHP who has an office on the floor below, and the patient begins therapy the following week. The doctor and MHP have regularly scheduled calls to check in about shared patients. On these calls, the doctor updates the MHP on which patients seem to need the most attention and what is happening with their treatment, and the MHP adjusts the patient's therapy treatment plan accordingly.
4. Close collaboration in a partly integrated system	Providers share the same sites and have some systems in common; there are regular interactions about patients, coordinated treatment plans, shared allegiance to a biopsychosocial paradigm, and a basic understanding and appreciation of each other's roles. Pragmatics may still be difficult, however, with some operational discrepancies, occasional team meetings, and unresolved tensions over the physician's greater power.	The REI refers patient directly to the staff MHP, who meets with patient in their next available opening. The REI communicates concerns to the MHP via notes and a quick face-to-face check in. They agree that the MHP will work with the patient to develop strategies to cope with distress. As treatment continues, the nurses and doctors refer the patient back to the MHP when the patient voices distress. The staff are appreciative that the MHP is there to support the patient, but feel irritated with the demands this patient is placing on them.

Table 6.1 (cont.)

Level	Description	Example: *REI clinic is treating a patient who is showing symptoms of depression . . .*
5. Close collaboration in a fully integrated system	Providers share the same site and the same systems; all are committed to a biopsychosocial systems paradigm and have an in-depth understanding of each other's roles. Regular, collaborative team meetings are held to discuss patient issues and team collaboration issues, and conscious efforts are made to balance power among providers, according to patient needs and provider expertise.	The REI refers patient directly to the staff MHP, who meets with the patient in their next available opening. The REI communicates concerns to the MHP via notes and a quick face-to-face check in. Together, they agree that the patient is distressed and discuss therapy goals. The MHP notices from notes the patient is emailing staff almost every day. The MHP checks in with nursing staff at a team meeting, who acknowledge frustrations as this patient never seems satisfied. The MHP helps reframe the pattern: the patient is sad and scared, which is driving the emails. The nurses are able to view the patient more sympathetically. Together, the team creates a plan for addressing patient questions; this reduces the burden on any one staff member and improves communication with the patient.

Adapted from Doherty[23] and McDaniel, Doherty, and Hepworth[1]. This table presents an example related to integration of mental health services. The same concepts would apply to other services (e.g., nutrition counselors, CAM providers).

for patients who are already feeling depressed, overwhelmed, or hopeless. Therefore, clinics adopting a collaborative care model will need to be cognizant of these potential issues to make sure that patients' psychosocial needs are being appropriately addressed.

Integrative Care

At levels 4 and 5, services are embedded together on site and are integrated to varying degrees. These integrative models may provide significant benefits. For example, having MHPs and other providers embedded within the treatment system means they will be more immediately available to provide counseling to patients (and to staff), they can communicate seamlessly with the rest of the treatment team, and their presence conveys to the patient that clinic is offering a more holistic model of healthcare[8]. This structure can also serve to communicate to patients that physical and behavioral health are interdependent and are both priorities of the clinic[26]. Further, and perhaps most critically, this model has the potential to reduce barriers to the very type of supportive services that will potentially improve fertility potential and reduce treatment dropout.

There is no single way that an integrative care system is set up, but there are common elements. In addition to sharing space and systems, providers will share expectations for team-based prevention and treatment. They will communicate regularly about patients and about clinic processes, and they will value the different perspective and skills that each set of providers bring to the table[1]. In the words of Doherty: "It deals adequately with the most difficult and complex biopsychosocial cases that present challenging management problems. This is a team that can contain its anxiety and do something constructive with it[23]."

Beyond these common aims, integrated services can be delivered in a variety of formats. For example, both the University of California, San Francisco (UCSF) Center for Reproductive Health and the Northwestern Fertility and Reproductive Medicine clinic currently have teams of MHPs on staff. At UCSF, a psychological consultation is required for certain patient groups (e.g., those using a known donor, an egg donor, or surrogacy); for others, a meeting with a psychologist is typically recommended but optional. Patients who report distress to their doctor or nurses will get referred to one of the psychologists or to the staff psychiatrist. This targeted approach aims to deliver the services of the MHP team to those patients who need it most, thereby conserving resources and focusing efforts on the patients most in need of psychoeducation and support. Conversely, at Northwestern, every patient is required to meet with a staff psychologist before their first treatment cycle. This preventive approach aims to enable the team to address whatever questions and concerns a patient might have at the outset, thereby preempting difficulties that might otherwise arise later in treatment. It further makes sure that every patient is connected with an MHP, thus making it much easier to reach out if needs arise during the course of treatment.

Another more comprehensive example of integrative care can be found at Boston IVF (BIVF)[8]. This clinic houses the Domar Center for Mind/Body Health. The Domar Center is integrated with BIVF services and shares systems, but operates within its own space. The center has a team of psychologists who provide a similar set of services to those at UCSF. In addition, the psychologists provide a free 30-minute counseling session to any patient who wants it after any failed treatment cycle and are available "on call" to help patients in crisis. In addition, the Domar Center offers an array of other services directly on site: nutrition counseling, acupuncture, and a 10-week mind/body program. The BIVF clinic also has a team of social work counselors who specialize in helping patients navigate third-party services (e.g., donor sperm or egg, surrogacy) and make treatment-related decisions. The psychologists and social workers work together with the medical team to make patient care decisions.

The BIVF model also illustrates how the integrative approach can benefit not just patients but also the staff. The MHPs keep the staff up to date on mental-health-related research. They also attend team meetings and conduct regular "stress lunches," where the staff can consult with MHPs on strategies for managing challenging cases[8]. Staff members are encouraged to utilize the Domar Center services (e.g., crisis counseling, acupuncture) as needed. By providing education, training, and support to the whole staff, MHPs and other integrative members of the team have the potential to enhance the overall functioning of the clinic by helping to reduce staff stress and improving overall psychosocial patient care[10].

While the benefits of integrative care may be evident, this model also comes with its own considerations. First, providing integrative care requires a significant investment in infrastructure (e.g., space, equipment, record-keeping systems). Such a setup must be a financially and logistically viable option for the clinic. The financial impact may not be as daunting a prospect as it initially seems. If the integration of supportive services can indeed keep patients from dropping out of treatment and reduce staff burnout/costly turnover (see Chapter 12), the clinic stands to generate significantly more revenue. Thus, clinics should carefully evaluate the cost benefits before ruling out a move toward integrative care as too expensive.

Second, a clinic must be able to find providers willing to embrace an integrative approach, and the physician and staff leaders within the clinic must be committed to putting in the necessary effort to make it work. For example, medical providers must be willing to expand their perspective on patient care and consider how psychosocial considerations fit into the treatment plan. Conversely, MHPs, nutritionists, and CAM providers must become knowledgeable about infertility and fertility treatment services (e.g., terminology, diagnoses, and treatment options), and keep this knowledge base up to date as the field advances. They must further be able to deliver evidence-based interventions that flexibly fit the patient population needs, the time constraints, and the service delivery model of the clinic[27]. Bridging all these demands can be a tall order, and it can be difficult to find staff with appropriate training who can effectively function in this multifaceted way.

Finally, it is worth noting that some patients may prefer supportive services to be located outside of the REI clinic. If a patient experiences treatment failures, or has encountered difficult interactions with staff, returning to the clinic for counseling or acupuncture may be stressful or even retraumatizing. Additionally, when MHPs work for the clinic, it may make it harder for patients to be honest about how they are feeling (particularly if they are having negative feelings about the medical providers). In some cases, supportive services may be best delivered away from the source of the stress.

Tailoring the Approach

This chapter has primarily focused on how REI clinics can integrate dietary, behavioral, psychosocial, and alternative interventions with medical treatment. Different patients will have different needs, and clinics may need to collaborate with those who can provide additional skills and resources. Even a clinic that has achieved a "level 5" integration of care may need to reach outside to collaborate with other providers in certain situations. As illustrated in Figure 6.1, clinics often will need to use a hybrid of integrative and collaborative approaches to cover patient needs.

As an example, clinics are now serving a higher number of cancer patients. Historically, pregnancy after cancer diagnosis and treatment was rare. But today, with advances in cancer care and fertility preservation (FP) capabilities (see Chapter 10), patients often have options available for future family building. Clinics will interact with patients at different stages of their illness – a patient may present immediately after diagnosis for FP services, or they may return later for treatment using preserved gametes or donor gametes. REI clinic providers will need to coordinate care with the oncology

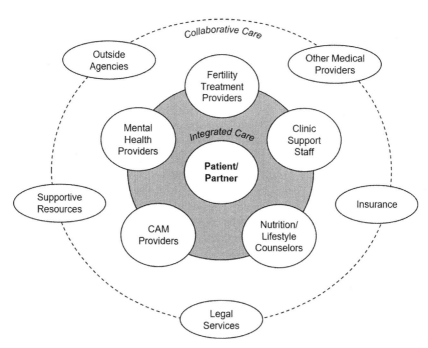

Figure 6.1 Ecosystem of integrative care. This figure shows an example of the ecosystem of fertility treatment care providers that may be found in integrative care. The figures at the center of the gray circle are the providers who might be located within an REI clinic who would work together to provide medical care and address psychological and socioemotional needs within an integrated treatment plan. Along the periphery are additional components, often external to the clinic, which may be required to meet a patient's family-building needs. This figure is not exhaustive, but rather illustrative of the complexities of needs that patients face as they navigate fertility treatment.

team, and will need to develop a knowledge base related to cancer care to effectively counsel patients on reproductive options.

Another growing population of patients are transgender patients and same-sex couples[28]. For transgender patients, providers will also need to be prepared to advise on FP options, and in some cases they may need to coordinate with primary care doctors on the management of hormone therapy during the course of fertility treatment. With regard to same-sex couples, clinic staff should be aware that these patients often face additional family-building challenges, such as access to insurance coverage and securing legal rights for both partners to the offspring. For example, even if two women are married and are allowed to have both their names on the birth certificate, it is still recommended that the nonbirth partner complete a formal adoption or judgment of parentage. Clinics will benefit from developing consultative relationships with family planning attorneys in their jurisdiction so they can best advise patients and direct them to appropriate legal resources.

The list of additional possible collaborative care providers is extensive. All clinics will work with outside agencies, such as sperm banks, egg banks, and those providing surrogacy services. REI clinics need to collaborate with doctors to manage any number of medical conditions. It is particularly necessary to develop relationships with psychiatrists who are comfortable managing medications during the perinatal period. Clinics may also need to be able to work in close concert with various insurance systems. Cost can be one of the greatest stressors of the treatment process, and clinic staff need to be able to help patients understand the costs and access coverage. For lower income patients, they may also want to establish relationships with institutions that may provide assistance in the form of grants or low-cost cycles. Some cases bring up complex legal or ethical issues – clinics need to know with whom to consult to make sure that their patients (and the clinic) are making sound decisions.

The integrative care components covered so far focus on the needs of the patient during treatment. Looking forward, clinics may also want to think about integrating services to support patients prior to and after treatment. Gameiro and colleagues[14] have observed that it would be useful for people to start thinking about their parenthood goals at an earlier age, and to understand the factors that could get in the way of these goals (e.g., age, sexually transmitted diseases, smoking). They suggest that fertility treatment providers can work to disseminate information to other stakeholders who might interface with people at these earlier stages of family planning (e.g., family planning associations, scientific societies) so prospective parents can do a better job planning ahead and protect their fertility potential. It may also be valuable for clinics to consider how to continue to support patients after conception occurs. For example, clinics can consider how to provide longer-term services for families they helped to create. Parents might later have questions regarding how to talk to their child about how they were brought into the world, or offspring may want to discuss considerations in reaching out to their sperm or egg donor. Fertility clinics will benefit from expanding their view of the many important roles the clinic can play in family building[29].

Conclusion

Every diagnosis feels like a unique experience for the patient and his/her partner. They will work to wrap their minds around what the diagnosis means for them, and they will have their own set of thoughts, feelings, and behaviors related to the diagnosis. But despite the fact that the experience feels deeply personal, many feel that they are treated as "just another patient[1]." This is why REI clinics will benefit from delivering integrative, patient-centered care that recognizes the complex biopsychosocial needs of patients. Integrative care can take different forms, and clinics will need to assess the level of integration that fits best. Clinics able to move toward an integrative model of care are positioned to realize a number of benefits. Integrative care brings together a team of providers who can contribute different perspectives, share the management of patient care, and optimize clinic functioning. This approach should result in less distress for patients, better long-term health, and more satisfaction with services for both patients and staff[14]. By taking a holistic view of patients' needs and delivering services that match, clinics will be positioned to support patients through treatment and help them make the decisions that feel right for themselves and for their future families.

Recommended Reading

Domar AD (2015). Creating a Collaborative Model of Mental Health Counseling for the Future. *Fertil Steril.* 104(**2**): 277–80.

Gameiro S, Boivin J, Domar A. Optimal in Vitro Fertilization in 2020 Should Reduce Treatment Burden and Enhance Care Delivery for Patients and Staff. *Fertil Steril.* 2013. 100 (**2**): 302–9.

McDaniel, SH, Doherty, WJ, & Hepworth, J. *Medical family therapy and integrated care (2nd Edition)*. Washington, DC: American Psychological Association; 2015.

References

1. McDaniel SH, Doherty WJ, Hepworth J. *Medical family therapy and integrated care (2nd Edition)*. Washington, DC: American Psychological Association; 2015.

2. Engel GL. The Need for a New Medical Model: A Challenge for Biomedicine. *Science*. 1977; 196: 129–36.

3. Academic Consortium for Integrative Medicine and Health. (2018). Definition of Integrative Medicine and Health. Website. https://imconsortium.org/about/mission/

4. Blount A. Integrated Primary Care: Organizing the Evidence. *Fam Syst Health*. 2003; 21: 121–33.

5. Rakel D, Weil A Philosophy of Integrative Medicine. In: Rakel D (ed.) *Integrative Medicine* (4th Edition). Philadelphia, PA: Elsevier; 2018: 2–11.

6. Domar AD, Zuttermeister PC, Friedman R. The Psychological Impact of Infertility: A Comparison with Patients with Other Medical Conditions. *J Psychosom Obstet Gynaecol*. 1993; 14 Suppl: 45–52.

7. Holley SR, Pasch LA, Bleil ME, Gregorich S, Katz PK, Adler NE. Prevalence and Predictors of Major Depressive Disorder for Fertility Treatment Patients and Their Partners. *Fertil Steril*. 2015; 103: 1332–9.

8. Domar AD. Creating a Collaborative Model of Mental Health Counseling for the Future. *Fertil Steril*. 2015; 104: 277–80.

9. Gameiro S, Boivin J, Peronace L, Verhaak CM. Why Do Patients Discontinue Fertility Treatment? A Systematic Review of Reasons and Predictors of Discontinuation in Fertility Treatment. *Hum Reprod Update*. 2012; 18: 652–69.

10. Grill E. Role of the Mental Health Professional in Education and Support of the Medical Staff. *Fertil Steril*. 2015; 104: 271–6.

11. Klock SC. When Treatment Appears Futile: The Role of the Mental Health Professional and End-of-Treatment Counseling. *Fertil Steril*. 2015; 104: 267–70.

12. Frederiksen Y, Farver-Vestergaard I, Skovgard NG, Ingerslev HJ, Zachariae R. Efficacy of Psychosocial Interventions for Psychological and Pregnancy Outcomes in Infertile Women and Men: A Systematic Review and Meta-Analysis. *BMJ Open*. 2015; 5: e006592.

13. Boivin J, Gameiro S. Evolution of Psychology and Counseling in Infertility. *Fertil Steril*. 2015; 104: 251–9.

14. Gameiro S, Boivin J, Domar A. Optimal in Vitro Fertilization in 2020 Should Reduce Treatment Burden and Enhance Care Delivery for Patients and Staff. *Fertil Steril*. 2013; 100: 302–9.

15. Norman RJ, Mol BWJ. Successful Weight Loss Interventions Before in Vitro Fertilization: Fat Chance? *Fertil Steril*. 2018; 110: 581–6.

16. Rodino IS, Byrne SM, Sanders KA. Eating Disorders in the Context of Preconception Care: Fertility Specialists' Knowledge, Attitudes, and Clinical Practices. *Fertil Steril*. 2017; 107: 494–501.

17. Rooney KL, Domar AD. The Impact of Lifestyle Behaviors on Infertility Treatment Outcome. *Curr Opin Obstet Gynecol*. 2014; 26: 181–5.

18. National Center for Complementary and Integrative Health. (2018). Complementary, Alternative, or Integrative Health: What's in a Name? Online article. https://nccih.nih.gov/health/integrative-health.

19. Boivin J, Schmidt L. Use of Complementary and Alternative Medicines Associated with a 30% Lower Ongoing Pregnancy/Live Birth Rate During 12 Months of Fertility Treatment. *Hum Reprod*. 2009; 24: 1626–31.

20. Zheng CH, Huang GY, Zhang MM, Wang W. Effects of Acupuncture on Pregnancy Rates in Women Undergoing in Vitro Fertilization: A Systematic Review and Meta-Analysis. *Fertil Steril*. 2012; 97: 599–611.

21. Domar AD, Gross J, Rooney K, Boivin J. Exploratory Randomized Trial on the Effect of a Brief Psychological Intervention on Emotions, Quality of Life, Discontinuation, and Pregnancy Rates in in Vitro Fertilization Patients. *Fertil Steril.* 2015; 104: 440–51.

22. Peloquin K, Brassard A, Arpin V, Sabourin S, Wright J. Whose Fault Is It? Blame Predicting Psychological Adjustment and Couple Satisfaction in Couples Seeking Fertility Treatment. *J Psychosom Obstet Gynaecol.* 2018; 39: 64–72.

23. Doherty WJ. The Whys and Levels of Collaborative Family Health Care. *Fam Syst Med.* 1995; 13: 275–81.

24. Foy R, Hempel S, Rubenstein L, Suttorp M, Seelig M, Shanman R et al. Meta-Analysis: Effect of Interactive Communication Between Collaborating Primary Care Physicians and Specialists. *Ann Intern Med.* 2010; 152: 247–58.

25. van Orden M, Hoffman T, Haffmans J, Spinhoven P, Hoencamp E. Collaborative Mental Health Care Versus Care As Usual in a Primary Care Setting: A Randomized Controlled Trial. *Psychiatr Serv.* 2009; 60: 74–9.

26. Poleshuck EL, Woods J. Psychologists Partnering with Obstetricians and Gynecologists: Meeting the Need for Patient-Centered Models of Women's Health Care Delivery. *Am Psychol.* 2014; 69: 344–54.

27. McDaniel SH, Grus CL, Cubic BA, Hunter CL, Kearney LK, Schuman CC et al. Competencies for Psychology Practice in Primary Care. *Am Psychol.* 2014; 69: 409–29.

28. Holley SR, Pasch LA. Counseling Lesbian, Gay, Bisexual, and Transgender Patients. In: *Fertility counseling: clinical guide and case studies.* Cambridge, UK: Cambridge University Press. 2015; 180–96.

29. Pasch LA, Pasch Lauri A. New Realities for the Practice of Egg Donation: A Family-Building Perspective. *Fertil Steril.* 2018; 110: 1194–202.

Psychological Counseling: Ethical Challenges of the Future

Elizabeth Grill and Lindsay Childress-Beatty

Introduction

The interplay between psychological and ethical issues continues to shape and define the role and responsibilities of professionals in the field of ART. Advances in ART have brought the process of creating a child some distance from nature, enabling physicians to offer patients a variety of permutations in terms of conceiving and carrying offspring. Women can be stimulated to produce multiple oocytes, resulting in multiple births that would not otherwise have occurred. Patients can receive donor gametes – eggs and/or sperm or embryos – to create children who (from a genetic point of view) would not otherwise have been created and whose genetic makeup does not reflect their own. Patients can freeze gametes for future family building that challenge the parameters of natural reproductive ability and can even be used posthumously.

Professionals are ethically challenged to stay informed about rapidly changing medical treatments and technologies to help patients understand and navigate medical systems and make informed decisions about their reproductive care. Ethical issues that once required psychological consultation such as multifetal pregnancy reduction and embryo disposition are becoming less problematic with the global shift to single ETs and offerings of oocyte cryopreservation, which allow women to freeze their gametes without creating embryos. Oocyte cryopreservation brings its own new ethical quandaries. The overlap between ethical dilemmas, how patients psychologically experience these issues, and the ethical positions of clinics and practitioners, are a part of the ongoing relationships and responsibilities of professionals in the field.

Reproductive technology has a wide-ranging impact on donors, gestational carriers, offspring, current and future siblings, as well as the family, community, and health systems. Professionals must consider the patient(s) sitting in front of them as well as the impact of their work on all these additional affected parties and the various levels of ethical duty owed to each[1]. The MHP trained in the area of fertility counseling is the best option to help clients and practitioners consider the psychosocial issues and ethical dilemmas generated by the vast array of treatment possibilities. This work requires a multidisciplinary approach to treatment and counseling, which includes medical, psychosocial, legal, and ethical considerations, including the best interests of the patients, donors, carriers, and potential offspring.

The Integration of the MHP in ART

The MHP is in the forefront of the trend toward interdisciplinary teams in medicine integrating psychosocial issues into medical decision-making as well as patient-centered care[2,3]. The value of the MHP within the reproductive medicine field has long been recognized with MHPs participating in ethics committees and helping with controversial decisions[4].

ASRM and ESHRE[5,6,7,8] have issued several ethics statements and practice guidelines addressing current ethical issues in ART. Many of these statements explicitly recommend that patients meet with an MHP trained in infertility counseling and that clinics consult with an MHP as part of their multidisciplinary team to discuss the many complicated ethical and psychosocial issues related to their reproductive care.

Globally, the status of infertility counseling with regard to mandating counseling and defining the MHP role is uneven. For example, some jurisdictions in Australia, New Zealand, and the UK have professional guidelines that both mandate and prescribe infertility counseling, while in other areas, professional guidelines are produced by infertility counseling organizations but have less influence[9]. Although MHPs are an integral part of clinics and fertility, and endorsed by governing bodies such as the ASRM and ESHRE, international support for psychosocial counseling is still needed to emphasize its importance in conjunction with ART.

Guiding Principles of Practice

Ethics codes of medical and MHPs provide an ethical framework, but do not provide precise guidance concerning practice within an interdisciplinary team or particular reproductive clinical situations. The ASRM and ESHRE ethics statements, as well as general principles of bioethics, must also guide the professionals' decision-making. In addition, human rights and social justice concepts increasingly play a role in ethical decision-making.

One of the most fundamental ethical debates in reproductive medicine is whether ART involves unnatural practices. The development of IVF has made it possible for one child to have as many as five different "parents" including an ovum donor, a sperm donor, a gestational carrier, and the two rearing parents. Furthermore, the technology exists for the intended parents to select the sex of the child and even specific genetic characteristics. Successful cryopreservation of sperm, embryos, and most recently oocytes, has enabled people to preserve their potential fertility almost indefinitely. These parental configurations raise profoundly difficult and often disturbing ethical questions and have forced the people working in the field of ART to confront whether specific technologies should be used for assisted reproduction simply because they exist.

Many experts in the field argue for procreative liberty, asserting that since the Constitution of the United States affords people the right to procreate on their own, it also gives individuals that right with assistance. Some argue that helping couples to become parents using reproductive technology supports autonomy, beneficence, and justice: three of the four ethical principles foundational to modern United States medical ethics[10]. Similar ethical arguments also support planned oocyte cryopreservation by women in an attempt to preserve future parenthood[11]. Autonomy, as well as the human rights concept of the right to a private family life, is supported when couples are given the power to make decisions regarding their treatment based on all the information pertaining to their own situation. Beneficence is furthered when couples are able to achieve their long-sought-after goal of parenthood. Justice exists if all who are in need can utilize the technology; although for some, the rising cost of treatment and the lack of insurance coverage in many states may impede justice and can be viewed as a social justice issue. At times, autonomy may also collide with nonmaleficence, the fourth ethical principle, especially when a patient requests a particular treatment that his/her provider believes may do harm to the patient or potential child. In these cases, one principle must be compromised for the sake of the other. Furthermore, what is ethical may vary depending on the social, spiritual, and religious community from which one arises and in which one chooses to raise a family[12]. In helping the parties navigate the profound ethical questions involved in ART, professionals must consider the impact on intended parents, offspring, involved donor(s) or gestational carrier, and any relevant cultural communities, as well as the impact of the specific ART on the larger society.

Defining the Role of Professionals in ART

Defining and shaping the role of professionals in ART has been the subject of ethical debate from the beginning. There is inherent tension between those who view their role as gatekeepers and those who define their role as counselors and educators providing support and psychoeducation. Considerable literature has addressed the ethical dilemmas faced by MHPs themselves in their complex roles[13].

Procreative libertarians believe in patient autonomy. Proponents feel that people have the right to procreate and parent, and therefore the role of professionals is to provide support, education, preparation, and treatment, but not to determine which patients are psychologically eligible for treatment or fit to parent[14]. Procreative libertarians differ from those who view the role as gatekeeper. Gatekeepers believe that the medical and psychological teams have the responsibility to consider the risks and prohibit treatment in situations that could potentially cause harm to the patient, recipient, donor, carrier, or unborn child. Gatekeepers believe to fail to act on the best interests of the patients and children would be in violation of the ethical principle of beneficence. Some experts also argue that social justice and human rights principles require consideration of potential exploitation of donors and gestational carriers, in addition to intended parents and offspring[15].

Regardless of the role the ART professional chooses or is asked to perform, all staff must clearly define their role to patients and clinics to minimize misunderstanding. Professionals must make it clear whether they are functioning in the role of the psychoeducational consultant or evaluator/gatekeeper and clarify any misconceptions about their role. Patients should understand exactly what information, if any, will be kept confidential and what information will be shared with the treatment team, partner, or other family members. *If the professional chooses to act as gatekeeper, he/she must clearly disclose the evaluation process to patients in advance of any discussions so that patients can choose if and how to proceed.* The varying roles of the ART professional will inevitably continue to be a major discussion point within the field[14].

Withholding Treatment

While historically physicians have an obligation to honor refusals of treatment, they do not have an obligation to honor all requests for treatment. Physicians may deny treatment based on the potential risks to the patient, donor, or carrier, and even risks to the prospective offspring.

Practitioners are often confronted with patients who do not appear capable of providing the necessary care for a child. Future offspring are entitled to a safe home and minimally competent childrearing. These interests must be weighed against the desires and rights of the intended parents to receive the treatment they need to reproduce and the provider's own sense of moral responsibility in deciding which patients to treat. While most will agree about extreme situations involving physical or sexual abuse, psychological instability, or addiction presenting risks to the child's well-being, it is more difficult to determine what good-enough parenting is without running the risk of being discriminatory[14].

The ASRM Ethics Statement and ESHRE Task Force on Ethics and Law set forth guidelines for childrearing ability and the provisions of fertility services[5,8], and indicate that fertility programs may withhold services from prospective patients on the basis of well-substantiated judgments that the intended parent(s) would be unable to provide adequate childcare and/or are likely to cause significant harm to a future child. The Ethics Statement is clear that programs should not discriminate against persons with disabilities nor violate that person's constitutional rights. However, practitioners could potentially refuse to treat based on uncontrolled or untreated psychiatric problems, substance abuse, violent or criminal behavior, child or ongoing partner abuse, and previous loss of parental rights.

Assessing parental fitness presents numerous challenges because of the many interests that are involved and because there are no reliable methods to predict who will become a good parent. This decision should only be rendered after thorough multidisciplinary investigation. For example, medical staff are often quick to assume that a history or current episode of psychiatric problems automatically disqualify that patient from being a capable intended parent. The person's history, compliance with treatment plan, and current level of functioning must be evaluated prior to a determination. The ethical practitioner bases decisions on scientific and professional knowledge, and has an adequate basis for professional opinions. Often, the decision does not require a refusal to treat the patient but rather the recommendation to seek the necessary help prior to a future reevaluation with collaboration and consultation with the patient's outside treatment team. The Ethics Statement makes clear that, because it is so difficult to judge the potential risk to the unborn child(ren), fertility providers are not ethically obligated to refuse services in all cases in which there might be a question about such risk.

Third-Party Reproduction

The use of a third party to form families and the involvement of MHPs is now well established, and the number of children born each year to parents using egg or sperm donation and gestational carriers is growing. The donors, recipients, carriers, and off-spring, as well as the programs that manage their care, all have distinct but at times competing interests, rights, and obligations. Psychological evaluation and counseling by a qualified MHP are strongly recommended for gamete and embryo donors and carriers, along with psychological consultation for recipients and their partners, if applicable. The assessment should include a psychosocial interview and, where appropriate, psychological testing. In cases of directed donation, the potential impact of the relationship between the donor and recipient should be explored, as well as potential psychological risks, evidence of coercion, and any plans that may exist relating to disclosure and future contact[16].

The Donors

Since technology has made it possible to separate the various components of mother-hood, ovum donors and/or surrogates are subjected to medical and psychological risks not leading to their own parenting. Experts question whether donors, especially those who have not yet experienced parenthood, truly understand the long-term emotional implications of their donation. Many argue that those who are infertile have the right to choose a procedure with potential physical and psychological harm, but that it is morally unacceptable to subject a young, fertile woman to these same risks when she is not the intended parent[12]. According to the ASRM Ethics Committee[17] and ESHRE Task Force on Ethics and Law[7], programs have a duty to inform donors, as well as recipients of donor gametes, about potential legal, medical, and emotional issues involved in donation.

ART professionals should play an active part in helping donors contemplate whether they are certain that their reasons for undertaking donation are right for them now and in the future. They must give serious thought to how they feel about donating their genetic material to help create a child that they may or may not have future contact with. They must understand the differences between the genetic, gestational, and rearing aspects of motherhood. Those who have not started or completed their families must imagine how they would feel about having genetic children in the world should they become infertile themselves. Donors must understand the limitations of anonymity and consider their feelings regarding not knowing whether a child(ren) was created with their help and any likelihood of future contact.

Family Donation

Gamete donation has made it possible for participants to cross generational lines, raising many complicated ethical issues. The reasons for seeking a familial donor or surrogate are varied. Some prefer familial donation to preserve the family's genetic heritage. For others, choosing a family member could reduce costs or speed up the process that can often involve months of waiting for a donor or surrogate. These arrangements may occur intragenerationally between siblings or cousins or intergenerationally when a parent donates to a child, a mother gestates her daughter's embryo, or a child donates to a parent. The importance of the goal to preserve genetic linkages may be questioned when the reproductive arrangements become so extraordinary and complex.

While familial arrangements may offer advantages over the use of anonymous donors and surrogates, they also present unique counseling challenges. Intrafamilial collaborative reproduction raises ethical concerns distinct from other ART arrangements. The appearance of incest (i.e., sexual relations between two related individuals) or consanguinity (i.e., reproduction between individuals who are closely related genetically) are issues raised by the ASRM Ethics Committee. There are also obvious concerns about undue influence to participate, and possible confused parentage for resulting children [17,18,19]. For example, a brother may not provide sperm to fertilize a sister's eggs or a sister provide eggs to be fertilized by a brother's sperm. Similarly, a father should not provide the sperm to replace that of his daughter's infertile husband. Nor should a mother provide eggs to replace those of her son's infertile wife.

Cases without genetic connection that give the appearance of incest or consanguinity have the potential to cause emotional harm to the donor, surrogate, offspring, and extended family, but should not automatically be barred[19]. For example, a sister may donate eggs for her brother's infertile wife to be inseminated by donor sperm or a brother may provide sperm to a sister who uses anonymous egg donation. Professionals recommend careful medical and psychological counseling to all of the parties involved so that coercion is avoided and the potential medical and psychological risks are thoroughly considered. ART practitioners must look for coercion where one party feels obligated to the other and sometimes need to help one party decline an uncomfortable request.

In child-to-parent donations, professionals must address the imbalance of power and the inherent boundary violations that may leave the family system or individual relationships vulnerable and at risk. The Ethics Committee notes that adult child-to-parent arrangements require caution to avoid coercion, and parent-to-adult child arrangements are acceptable in limited situations. Some experts argue that, because most children feel indebted to some degree, they are not truly free to say no to their parent's request[20]. For example, how will it appear to the participants and a potential child when a mother remarries and wants to use her daughter as the donor? ART practitioners must consider the daughter's relationship with the stepparent to make sure that there are no sexual overtones. The daughter may be financially or otherwise dependent on her mother and stepfather and may therefore feel obligated or coerced. In addition, the donor's father will be the genetic grandfather of his ex-wife's child with her new husband. Finally, she may have some conflicting feelings about being both biological mother and sister to this child. It is critical for all the parties involved to have a clear understanding of boundaries and to think through scenarios that may challenge these arrangements in the future. Some professionals feel supportive of a parent donating to a son or in some cases to a daughter, because the parent–child relationship includes the concept of a parent giving to their child.

The ASRM Ethics Committee[17] and ESHRE Task Force on Ethics and Law[18] suggests that the use of adult intrafamilial gamete donors and gestational surrogates is generally ethically acceptable in some situations and in some conditions when all participants are fully informed and counseled. ART practitioners must help all the parties explore their motivations, concerns, expectations, wants, hopes, and fears regarding the process. The psychosocial impact on the potential children and their right to privacy requires special attention as well. Programs that participate in intrafamilial arrangements should develop policies for such procedures and be prepared to spend additional time counseling not only the intended parents, the gamete donors, and the gestational surrogates, but also their partners and children to ensure that they have made free, informed decisions[16,19]. All parties should be in agreement regarding disclosure to the potential child and otherwise. Ultimately, the donor should feel comfortable allowing the recipients to make all decisions related to disclosure, the pregnancy, and the potential child's upbringing. When the assessment reveals concerns about undue emotional or financial pressures on the prospective donor or surrogate, unhealthy family dynamics, or incest or consanguinity, the program is ethically justified in denying access to these procedures. They should also offer prospective donors and gestational surrogates the option of being excluded as participants without other family members learning of their reluctance to participate.

Information Sharing and Disclosure

Using a third-party donor or donor gametes involves a complicated interplay of psychosocial needs of the donor, recipient, carrier, and offspring, as well as program obligations. Programs should be aware of the complexities surrounding the often-competing interests with regard to information sharing in light of changing realities regarding anonymity [21].

Whether or not children conceived using donated gametes should be told about their genetic origins remains one of the most disputed ethical issues. The question of openness versus secrecy is a complicated one, involving profound ethical, legal, religious, and psychosocial issues. The historical trend of not encouraging disclosure to children or others has changed with the recognition of the hazards of secrecy[16] and the rights of children to know the identity of their genetic parents[22]. Support has grown for disclosing the fact of donation and allowing offspring access to nonidentifying donor information as evidenced by research showing an increase in the number of parents who intend to disclose[6].

There is an increasing opinion that it is not justifiable to keep such information secret based on arguments involving children's inherent right to know about their genetic/ gestational beginnings, the possible negative effect of secrecy on family relationships, and/or the accessibility of genetic information rendering secrets impossible[23]. For example, children are now asking parents for genetic testing as a holiday or birthday gift because their friends did it for fun. Donors, who at one point chose anonymity, later decide to do genetic testing or join a registry and reach out to offspring who share genetic links. A school science unit on genetics can lead to new questions from children conceived via donor eggs who are unaware of their origins. After comparing their eye color, blood type, and earlobe attachment to their parents', children may question why their results do not match their parents as they had been taught, leaving the parents wondering how to respond.

In 1984, Sweden was the first country to make donors non-anonymous by law. Several countries have since removed donor anonymity: Austria, Finland, Iceland, the Netherlands, Switzerland, the UK, New Zealand, and the Australian states of New South Wales, Victoria, and Western Australia[15]. Indeed, some argue that donor anonymity is anachronistic and contact with the donor should now be considered normative. For that reason, increased focus in counseling on preparing the intended parents for possible future contact with the donor is considered important when discussing family-building[24].

A child's request for available information concerning his or her non-anonymous donor requires that the parents have informed the child of their use of a donor. The ASRM Ethics Committee[22,6], other advisory groups, and researchers have encouraged recipient parent(s) to disclose the fact of gamete donation to offspring, and a number of clinics provide for some form of future contact between donor and offspring if the participants agree. Proponents of disclosure argue that nondisclosure violates the child's fundamental right to know about his/her origins and could potentially undermine the donor-conceived person's identity development[25]. The human rights argument centers on the right to identity included in the United Nations Convention on the Rights of the Child[26]. Arguably, open communication, as opposed to secrets within families, promotes healthy family functioning[27,28]. Research on families who have disclosed indicates that few have regrets and disclosure does not appear to injure the child. Some research suggests a positive effect on parent–child relationships in disclosing families [29]. Other proponents of disclosure emphasize the medical interests of the donor-conceived child. Future medical emergencies could lead to possible discovery of the absence of a genetic match to their mothers or fathers[6]. Disclosure can protect the offspring's interest in knowing their genetic heritage, in securing accurate information about potential health problems, and in making future medical decisions[30]. However, some studies of children who have not been informed show they are doing well developmentally and psychologically, and have not been harmed by nondisclosure[31,32]. There are as yet no long-term studies to support this theory and there are numerous anecdotal reports of children and adults inadvertently finding out, leading to significant psychological issues.

Ethical concerns continue to arise as potential methods of future contact between the parties become more accessible. Contact, both deliberate and unexpected, between donors and offspring is being facilitated and promoted through websites offering assistance to offspring in tracing their origins and connecting with others who share their genetics. Direct-to-consumer (DTC) genetic testing also enables individuals to discover information about their genetic ancestry. The increasing availability of DTC genetic testing will result in individuals unaware of their donor conception inadvertently discovering their origins and identifying their anonymous donors and others sharing their genetics[23,33]. All the parties must understand that the connection does not necessarily end with the donation or birth of a child. Given the variation in programs with regard to archiving and sharing information as well as advances in DNA tracing, donors should also fully understand that offspring or intended parents might contact them in the future even if they chose "anonymous" donation. Couples should be encouraged to think through unplanned disclosure and the child's access to information through the growing availability of the Internet, genetic testing, and DNA databases[34].

Experts agree that the more the recipient couple feels comfortable and prepared for this parenting option, the more likely it is that they will be fulfilled as parents and make decisions that are in the child's best interest. Counseling and informed consent about disclosure and information sharing are essential for donors and the intended parents[30]. Intended parents planning to disclose should pick an ART facility that matches their expectations regarding the amount of information gathered, updated over time, and disclosed to recipients. The Ethics Committee encourages ART programs; sperm, oocyte, and embryo banks; and donation programs to develop flexible policies to accommodate varying information-sharing preferences, and encourages the promotion of the off-spring's interests, while respecting the privacy and autonomy interests of donors and recipient parents. Programs should clearly inform donors, intended parents, and carriers before their participation about the information that will be shared as part of the screening process as well as in the future. Programs are also obligated to inform all parties that policies cannot be guaranteed if laws or individual circumstances change and the possibility exists of future contact from offspring. Legal aspects of sperm and ovum donation, including anonymity, could be challenged in the future, thereby changing the public climate of openness versus secrecy. Other countries already have, or have sought to establish, open donor registries to protect the rights of the potential child. The ASRM recommends[6] that programs should include discussion encouraging donors and recipients to authorize the disclosure of nonidentifying medical information and that donors should be encouraged to allow nonidentifying and/or personal contact in the future if the offspring and donor agree. It also supports the gathering and storage of medical and genetic history information that can be provided to offspring if they request[30].

There are arguments both for and against disclosure and each couple should be allowed to decide with the help of trained ART professionals which choice is best for them and their child(ren) within the context of these issues.

How Old Is Too Old to Participate in Infertility Treatment?

Medical, psychological, and ethical factors weigh heavily in the decision to have a child at any age. Reproductive technology that extends a women's reproductive life, such as oocyte donation and cryopreservation, has enabled many women past traditional reproductive age to conceive and carry a pregnancy to term. Another ethical quandary is whether limits should be recommended for the application of ART to postmenopausal women and/or older men with arguments concerning age minimums and maximums. Ethicists question how old is too old and who should determine that age. How do practitioners weigh the risks of pregnancy against the rights of a woman to choose treatment? In addition, what about the children who will be raised by older parents who will most likely have a lifespan shorter than younger parents[35]?

At present, guidelines regarding this extension of the normal reproductive age vary greatly and, in the United States, there is great disparity among programs accepting postmenopausal women into treatment. A statement from the ASRM Ethics Committee [36] asserted that advanced reproductive age (ARA) is a risk factor for pregnancy loss, fetal anomalies, stillbirth, and obstetric complications, and recommends a thorough medical evaluation to assess fitness for pregnancy before transferring embryos to any woman of advanced reproductive age (>45 years). The ASRM further states that, because of concerns related to the high-risk nature of pregnancy, as well as longevity and the need for adequate psychosocial supports for raising a child to adulthood, treatment of women over the age of 55 should generally be discouraged even when they have no underlying medical problems.

Argument Against Reproductive Rights for Older Women

Major arguments against oocyte donation to postmenopausal women are that it is unnatural to transcend one's biological reproductive limits and concerns about childrearing, longevity, and medical risks. Some feel that there are medical and psychological risks for both the older recipients and the potential children that far outweigh the benefits[35,37]. One of the most frequently raised concerns with older people using ART tends to be whether older women and men are being irresponsible or selfish based on the increased risk with older parents that the children will suffer the loss of one or both parents before reaching adulthood[37,38]. Parental loss is one of the most stressful life events for children or adolescents[37] and when that loss occurs in childhood the child is at risk for emotional and behavioral problems, and psychiatric disorders including anxiety, depression, post-traumatic stress disorder, alcoholism, and other drug abuse problems, social withdrawal, and lowered self-esteem. Further, children who have lost a parent, particularly a mother, report it as "the end of childhood[35]." Before the loss of a parent, the child may also be the caregiver of an older parent. Research shows that these caregivers are at risk for depression, anxiety, and behavioral problems and have less time for age-appropriate concerns such as school and friendships. Consequently, children in caregiver roles are at increased risk for dropping out of school[39,40]. Another issue that is raised is whether older parents will have enough energy or physical stamina to properly interact with young children.

Argument for Reproductive Rights for Older Women

The ASRM noted that arguments in favor of oocyte donation to postmenopausal women are based on societal practices, medical efficacy and safety, gender equality, and reproductive freedom.

Some consider age limits for people to become parents a form of ageism. Similarly, denying women an alternative for reproduction at ages equivalent to men is considered by some to be sexist and prejudicial, especially as women generally live longer than men do. Autonomy and procreative liberty arguably do not depend on age. Proponents also argue that individuals with life-limiting illnesses are not necessarily prohibited from reproduction based solely on their shortened life expectancy. It is deemed medically safe, in most cases, for postmenopausal women in good health to carry a child using a younger person's eggs. Furthermore, in many cultures including our society, it is not uncommon for children to be raised by grandparents in the parenting role. There is therefore no reason to assume either that older individuals, who in most cases are clearly motivated and may have economic stability and increased time, lack the physical and psychological stamina for raising children or that society will be harmed by allowing them to procreate. Some research shows that the potential for greater financial and emotional stability older parents may offer can be an advantage to children.

The ASRM Ethics Committee concludes that, given the possibility that postmenopausal reproduction may satisfy the strong desire for offspring, it would be wrong to deny women the use of donated oocytes or embryos solely because of their age. The ASRM recommends that prospective older parents should be counseled regarding short- and long-term parenting and childrearing issues specific to their age[36]. The age and health of the partner, if present, should also be considered in this discussion. The statement also notes that it is ethically permissible for programs to decline to provide treatment to women of ARA based on concerns over their health and well-being.

Telemental Health and Modern Technological Medicine

The increasing use of information technology has brought challenging new ethical issues for the ART practitioner. Patient interactions via technology with ART personnel are increasingly seen as an important aspect of patient communication and a consumer-driven, enhanced patient experience.

Interactive communication devices, such as multimedia platform decision aids, have the promise of addressing individual patient preferences in receiving and processing information and preparing the practitioner for further targeted discussions with each patient[41,42]. Telemonitoring, such as in-home sonography during stimulation cycles, may limit travel requirements for some patients[43]. Mobile apps and wearable devices will allow patients to track fertility and pregnancy[44]. Accurate home diagnostic testing of sperm via a smartphone could lead to increased patient satisfaction, empowerment, and efficiency[45]. Text messaging and other forms of electronic communication will allow patients to be in immediate contact with providers. Virtual-reality platforms will provide patients with practice experiences and help with decision-making[46]. The use of AI may replace practitioner decision-making in some situations and enhance patient counseling of options[47,48].

In addition to obtaining enough knowledge of new developments in reproductive medicine to become competent in helping patients manage their infertility experience, professionals will also confront use of these technologies within the ART practice[49]. Assessment, counseling, and treatment may increasingly be conducted via videoconferencing. Competence to use the technology with patients as well as technological competence will be increasingly important. The professional must consider security issues as well as plan for emergency support of distant patients. The practitioner will also be required to explain the limitations and risks of its use to patients, including regarding confidentiality[49,50,51]. Practitioners must continue to follow the code of ethics of their profession when implementing any technological innovation.

The professional will also need to navigate through ethical decisions concerning when technology is a useful adjunct or substitute to current practices and when it falls short of the needs of the patient for an in-person experience. For example, a practice may conduct some consultations via videoconference using a special room with state-of-the-art equipment and technical support personnel. The practice considers the service a growth opportunity as well as a benefit to patients, and many patients are appreciative of saving the time and expense of travel. However, the practice begins to realize that internet connections are more unstable in remote areas. Patients differ in levels of adherence to norms typical when meeting in person. Practitioners must verify identity and contend with unprofessional backdrops, such as bedrooms, intrusive noises, and frequent interruptions. A few patients even seem oblivious to confidentiality concerns despite the nature of the consult. The clinic determines that it must educate patients on the mode of service and plan for exigencies.

Technology holds the promise of reaching patients who would otherwise not be able to obtain the services of practitioners competent in ART due to location or other personal restrictions. However, it also may permit individuals without the requisite training to provide substandard care. Ethically, professionals must consider whether the use of the technology is for the benefit of the patient rather than the practitioner[51].

The pace of change continues to accelerate in the field of ART. Practitioners will continue to be challenged to make ethical decisions when confronted by new issues arising from advances in both ART and information technology. The continued emphasis on ethical decision-making will be reinforced by a greater focus on patient-centered care, social justice, the impact of actions on the community or communities, and the preservation of human rights.

The overlap between patients' perceptions and the ethical positions of clinics and practitioners are an ongoing part of the relationships and responsibilities between professionals, patients, and staff. When wading through the multitude of ethical dilemmas that arise in ART, it is important to consider a multidisciplinary approach to treatment and counseling. This approach includes psychosocial, legal, and ethical considerations, as well as the best interests of the patients, donors, carriers, and potential offspring. Ongoing research into the psychosocial aspects of infertility, treatment approaches, and the impact on offspring, as well as donors, gestational carriers, and recipients, will provide additional guidance in ethical decision-making. Ethical and psychosocial considerations will continue to provide a framework for navigating ART's future.

Disclaimer: This chapter does not constitute a formal interpretation of the APA Ethical Principles of Psychologists and Code of Conduct, nor any other official APA policies.

References

1. Fisher MA. Replacing "Who Is the Client?" with a Different Ethical Question. *Prof Psychol: Res and Practice.* 2009; 40: 1–7.

2. Domar, A. Creating a Collaborative Model of Mental Health Counseling for the Future. *Fertil Steril.* 2015; 104: 277–80.

3. Gameiro S, Boivin J, Domar A. Optimal In Vitro Fertilization in 2020 Should Reduce Treatment Burden and Enhance Care Delivery for Patients and Staff. *Fertil Steril.* 2013; 100: 302–9.

4. Grill, E. Role of the Mental Health Professional in Education and Support of the Medical Staff. *Fertil Steril.* 2015; 104(**2**): 271–6.

5. Ethics Committee of the American Society for Reproductive Medicine. Child-Rearing Ability and the Provision of Fertility Services: An Ethics Committee Opinion. *Fertil Steril.* 2017; 108: 944–7.

6. Ethics Committee of the American Society for Reproductive Medicine. Interests, Obligations, and Rights in Gamete and Embryo Donation: An Ethics Committee Opinion. *Fertil Steril.* 2019; 111: 664–70.

7. ESHRE Task Force on Ethics and Law. Gamete and Embryo Donation. *Human Reprod.* 2002; 17(**5**): 1407–8.

8. ESHRE Task Force on Ethics and Law 13: The Welfare of the Child in Medically Assisted Reproduction. *Human Reprod.* 2007; 22(**10**) 2585–8.

9. Blyth, E. Guidelines for Infertility Counselling in Different Countries: Is There an Emerging Trend? *Human Reprod.* 2012; 27: 2045–6.

10. Beauchamp TL, Childress, JF. Principles of Biomedical Ethics 6th Edition. New York, NY: Oxford University Press; 2009.

11. Ethics Committee of the American Society for Reproductive Medicine. Planned Oocyte Cryopreservation for Women Seeking to Preserve Future Reproductive Potential: An Ethics Committee Opinion. *Fertil Steril.* 2018; 110: 1022–8.

12. Grill E, Josephs L, Brisman M. Legal and Ethical Issues. In: Chan P (ed.) Reproductive Medicine Secrets. Philadelphia: Hanley & Belfus, Inc., Medical Publishers; 2004; 342–62.

13. Gordon EG, Barrow RG. Legal and Ethical Aspects of Infertility Counseling. In:

LH Burns, SN Covington (eds.) Infertility Counseling: A Compressive Handbook for Clinicians. New York: Parthenon; 1999; 491–512.

14. Horowitz JH, Galst JP, Elster N. Ethical Dilemmas in Fertility Counseling. Washington, DC: American Psychological Association; 2010.

15. Blyth E, Thorn P, Wischmann T. CBRC and Psychosocial Counselling: Assessing Needs and Developing an Ethical Framework for Practice. *Reprod BioMed Online.* 2011; 23: 642–51.

16. Practice Committee of the American Society for Reproductive Medicine. Recommendations for Gamete and Embryo Donation: A Committee Opinion. *Fertil Steril.* 2013; 99: 47–62.

17. Ethics Committee of the American Society for Reproductive Medicine. Using Family Members as Gamete Donors or Gestational Carriers. *Fertil Steril.* 2017; 107: 1136–42.

18. ESHRE Task Force on Ethics and Law. Intrafamilial Medically Assisted Reproduction. *Hum Reprod.* 2011; 26(3): 504–9.

19. Marshall LA. Intergenerational Gamete Donation: Ethical and Societal Implications. *Am J Obstet Gynecol.* 1998; 178: 1171–6.

20. Sureau C, Shenfield F. Oocyte Donation by a Daughter. *Hum Reprod.* 1995; 10: 1334.

21. Braverman AM, Schlaff WD. End of Anonymity: Stepping into the Dawn of Communication and a New Paradigm in Gamete Donor Counseling. *Fert Steril.* 2019; 111: 1102–3.

22. Ethics Committee of the American Society for Reproductive Medicine. Informing Offspring of Their Conception by Gamete or Embryo Donation: A Committee Opinion. *Fertil Steril.* 2018; 109: 601–5.

23. Borry P, Rusu O, Dondorp W, Wert G, Knoppers BM, Howard HC. Anonymity: Direct-to-Consumer Genetic Testing and Donor Conception. *Fertil Steril.* 2014; 101: 630–2.

24. Pasch LA. New Realities for the Practice of Egg Donation: A Family Building Perspective. *Fertil Steril.* 2018; 110: 1194–202.

25. Frith L. Gamete Donation and Anonymity: The Ethical and Legal Debate. *Hum Reprod.* 2001; 16: 818–24.

26. Lyons D. Domestic Implementation of the Donor-Conceived Child's Right to Identity in Light of the Requirements of the UN Convention on the Rights of the Child. *Int J Law Policy Fam.* 2018; 32: 1–26.

27. Hahn SJ, Craft-Rosenberg M. The Disclosure Decisions of Parents Who Conceive Children Using Donor Eggs. *J Obstet Gynecol Neonatal Nurs.* 2002; 31: 283–93.

28. Indekeu A, Dierickx K, Schotsmans P, Daniels KR, Rober P, D'Hooghe T. Factors Contributing to Parental Decision Making in Disclosing Donor Conception: A Systematic Review. *Hum Reprod Update.* 2013; 19: 714–33.

29. Golombok S, Readings J, Blake L, Casey P, Mellish L, Marks A, Jadva V. Children Conceived by Gamete Donation: Psychological Adjustment and Mother-Child Relationships at Age 7. *J Fam Psychol.* 2011; 25: 230–9.

30. Ravitsky V. Conceived and Deceived: The Medical Interests of the Donor Conceived. *Hastings Cent Rep.* 2012; 42: 17–22.

31. Ilioi EC, Golombok S. Psychological Adjustment in Adolescents Conceived by Assisted Reproduction Techniques: A Systematic Review. *Hum Reprod Update.* 2015; 21: 84–96.

32. Readings J, Blake L, Casey P, Jadva V, Golombok S. Secrecy, Disclosure and Everything In-Between: Decisions of Parents of Children Conceived by Donor Insemination, Egg Donation, and Surrogacy. Reprod Biomed Online 2011; 22: 485–95.

33. Su P. Direct-to-Consumer Genetic Testing: A Comprehensive View. *Yale J Biol Med.* 2013; 86: 359–65.

34. Klotz M. Wayward Relations: Novel Searches of the Donor-Conceived for Genetic Kinship. *Med Anthropol.* 2016; 365.

35. Zweifel, J. Donor Conception from the Viewpoint of the Child: Positives, Negatives, and Promoting the Welfare of the Child. *Fertil Steril.* 2015; 104: 513–19.

36. Ethics Committee of the American Society for Reproductive Medicine. Oocyte or Embryo Donation to Women of Advanced Reproductive Age. *Fertil Steril.* 2016; 106: e3–7.

37. Zweifel JE. Last Chance or Too Late? Counseling Prospective Older Parents. In: Covington SN (ed.) Fertility Counseling: Clinical Guide and Case Studies. New York: Cambridge University Press; 150–65.

38. Arias E, Xu J. United States Life Tables (2017). National Vital Statistics Reports 68 (7), June 24, 2019 (Tables A and B). Available at: http://www.cdc.gov/nchs/dat a/nvsr/nvsr68/nvsr07_508.pdf

39. Lackey NR, Gates MF. Adults' Recollections of Their Experiences as Young Caregivers of Family Members with Chronic Physical Illnesses. *J Adv Nurs.* 2001; 34: 320–8.

40. Bauman LJ, Foster G, Silver EJ, Berman R, Gamble I, Muchaneta L. Children Caring for Their Ill Parents with HIV/AIDS. *Vulnerable Child Youth Stud.* 2006; 1: 56–70.

41. Elster N. Enhancing Shared Decision Making in Assisted Reproductive Technologies through the Use of Multimedia Platforms for Informed Consent. *Fertil Steril.* 2018; 110: 1267.

42. Madeira JL, Rehbein J, Christianson MS, Lee M, Parry JP, Pennings G, Lindheim SR. Using the Engaged MD Multimedia Platform to Improve Informed Consent for Ovulation Induction, Intrauterine Insemination and in Vitro Fertilization. *Fertil Steril.* 2018; 110: 1338–46.

43. Gerris J. Telemonitoring in IVF/ICSI. *Curr Opin Gynecol Obstet.* 2017; 29: 160–7.

44. Goodale BM, Shilaih M, Falco L, Dammeier F, Hamvas G, Leensers B. Wearable Sensors Reveal Menses-Driven Changes in Physiology and Enable Prediction of the Fertile Window: Observational Study. *J Med Internet Res.* 2019; 21(**4**): e13404.

45. Agarwal A, Selvam MKP, Sharma R, Master K, Sharma A, Gupta S, Henkel R. Home Sperm Testing Device Versus Laboratory Sperm Quality Analyzer: Comparison of Motile Sperm Concentration. *Fertil Steril.* 2018; 110: 1277–84.

46. Palanica A, Docktor MJ, Lee A, Fossat Y. Using Mobile Virtual Reality to Enhance Medical Comprehension and Satisfaction in Patients and Their Families. *Perspect Med Ed.* 2019; 8: 123.

47. Tran A, Cooke S, Illingworth PJ, Gardner, DK. Artificial Intelligence as a Novel Approach to Embryo Selection. *Fertil Steril.* 2018; 110: e430.

48. Hunter Cohn K, Zhang Q, Copperman AB, Yurttas Beim P. Leveraging Artificial Intelligence for More Data-Driven Patient Counseling After Failed IVF Cycles. *Fertil Steril.* 2017; 108: e53-e54.

49. Joint Task Force for the Development of Telepsychology Guidelines for Psychologists. Guidelines for the Practice of Telepsychology. *Amer Psychol.* 2013; 68: 791–800.

50. National Association of Social Workers, Association of Social Work Boards, Council on Social Work Education, Clinical Social Work Association (2017). Standards for Technology in Social Work Practice (2017). Available at: http://www.socialworkers.org/includes/newIncl udes/homepage/PRA-BRO-33617.TechSt andards_FINAL_POSTING.pdf

51. The Ethics Committee of the American Society for Reproductive Medicine. Moving Innovation to Practice: A Committee Opinion. *Fertil Steril.* 2015; 104: 39–42.

Chapter 8

Using Technology to Enhance Communication in Medically Assisted Reproductive Care

Karin Hammarberg, Lone Schmidt, Gritt Malling, and Emily Koert

Introduction

Technology is increasingly used in all spheres of life, including in healthcare. In this chapter we summarize what is known about when and how technology can enhance communication in medically assisted reproduction (MAR) care and how this might improve the patient experience. While we found that technology benefits many aspects of MAR care and communication, others are better managed through compassionate and holistic person-to-person interaction.

When and How Technology Can Enhance MAR Care

There is robust evidence that women and men who use MAR to conceive want and place high value on staff who are professional, respectful, and empathetic in their interactions; who are knowledgeable and trustworthy and able to give personalized and evidence-based advice; and who involve both partners in the treatment process and decision-making. They also want written and verbal treatment information relevant to their unique circumstances and needs presented in a way they can understand and use to make informed treatment decisions[1]. There are many ways in which technology can be used to support clinic staff and patients and enhance communication in MAR care.

Making the Clinic's Website a Go-to Place for Comprehensive Information

The fertility clinic's website is its face to the world and great care should be taken to make it as user-friendly and informative as possible and to ensure it meets the information needs of the range of groups who might consider MAR. Patients who visit the website should be able to access comprehensive information about the credentials of the people who work at the clinic, the available treatment options and what they entail, evidence about the risks and benefits of the treatment options offered, age-specific success rates, cost of treatments, and what patients can do to improve their chance of success. Particular attention should be given to making information about chance of success as transparent and interpretable as possible, providing evidence for the benefits and risks of adjuvant therapies, and including information about and promoting preconception health optimization.

Communicating Chance of Success

Knowing what the chance is of having a baby as a result of treatment is of fundamental interest to those who consider MAR. But it can be difficult to understand information about success rates because it depends on how it is presented. Audits of clinic websites in the UK and Australia show that the quality of information about the chance of having a baby as a result of MAR is poor[2,3]. This is because most clinics define success as the chance of pregnancy per ET, which does not account for those who do not reach the ET stage or those who lose a pregnancy. Stating the proportion of women who have a baby after starting a stimulated cycle may allow a more realistic idea of what to expect. It may also be useful to quote the cumulative chance of having a baby after, e.g., three started stimulated cycles, including any frozen embryo transfers. This might help patients think of MAR as a series of treatments rather than a one off, which in turn may help them have more reasonable expectations and make them less likely to drop out of treatment if they are not successful the first time. Most importantly, since the woman's age is the greatest determinant of success, success rate figures should be age specific.

Benefits and Risks of Adjuvants

Increasingly clinics offer a range of adjuvant therapies to improve the chance of pregnancy including assisted hatching, time-lapse imaging, embryo "glue," sperm selection, immunotherapies, and others. For most adjuvants there is limited or no evidence about their effectiveness or potential risks[4,5]. At a minimum, clinic website information about adjuvants should include what is known about who they might benefit, how they might improve the chance of having a baby, what they cost, and what their risks are. In the absence of evidence, it should be stated that the possible benefits and risks of the adjuvant are unknown. While patients may be willing to try nonevidence-based treatments, their decisions should be well-informed.

Preconception Health Optimization

Evidence about the importance of intended parents optimizing their health before conception to improve their fertility, pregnancy health, and the health of the child at birth and in adulthood is growing[6]. Maternal and paternal obesity, poor nutrition, smoking, drug and alcohol use, and exposure to some environmental chemicals are all linked to poorer reproductive outcomes, including MAR outcomes. Patients seeking MAR are highly motivated to do what they can to improve their chance of having a baby and are likely to respond to preconception health optimization messages. Including information about the impact of lifestyle factors on MAR outcomes on clinic websites might prompt patients to commit to positive health behavior change and thereby

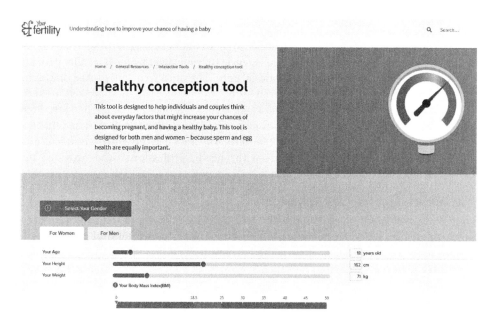

Figure 8.1 The Your Fertility preconception health self-assessment tool

improve their chance of conceiving and having a healthy baby. There are several emerging technology-based innovations to support positive health behaviors and preconception health optimization, including mobile phone apps and interactive web-based tools, which may help people seeking MAR[7,8]. Figure 8.1 shows an example of a web-based preconception health tool available on the "Your Fertility" website (www.yourfertility.org.au).

Technology to Enhance Patient Care

In day-to-day interactions with patients, all clinic staff are expected to provide patient-centered care, which is defined as care that is respectful of and responsive to individual patient preferences, needs, and values. For clinic staff to be able to provide optimal care, they need enabling clinic infrastructure. This includes an information technology system that: allows staff easy access to individual patient's records whenever they interact with them so that they can give personalized information and advice reflecting real-time results and outcomes; provides prompts when staff should consider proactively contacting the patient – e.g. after a failed cycle – and allows patients to communicate with staff when they need information or support.

Using Technology in Patient–Provider Communication

Electronic communication is convenient and time saving, and can facilitate patient–provider communication and information sharing. A survey among fertility patients in the United States showed that almost all were comfortable communicating electronically with the clinic and very few (<8%) had privacy concerns that prevented them from communicating electronically with their fertility doctor[9].

Written and verbal information about all aspects of MAR treatment provided by the clinic can be enhanced through an online forum where patients can access and communicate with clinic staff when they want and need to. In their analysis of the exchanges that occurred in one such forum, Aarts and colleagues[10] reported that most fertility patients gave more informational cues than emotional cues. The most frequently asked questions related to medication, factors associated with treatment success, and practical matters. The most common reason for asking questions online was that the patient had forgotten to ask these questions during their face-to-face visit. Almost all patients reported that the health professional had understood their question and had provided complete and reassuring responses. They also perceived the health professional who provided the responses as compassionate and respectful.

Using Technology to Provide Emotional Support

Some online interventions to support the emotional well-being of patients have been evaluated in RCTs, and findings suggest that they may be helpful and cost-effective complements to face-to-face counseling. Haemmerli and colleagues[11] evaluated a cognitive behavior coaching program for women and men in fertility treatment and found that the intervention significantly reduced the depression levels of clinically distressed and depressed patients. Cousineau and colleagues[12] tested a brief online education and support program for female infertility patients and reported that women in the intervention group felt significantly more informed about the medical decisions they made and had fewer infertility-related social concerns than women in the control group.

Using Technology to Monitor Quality of Care

Patient-reported experience measures (PREMs) are questionnaires assessing patients' perceptions of their experience while receiving care and are indicators of quality of care[13]. PREMs are increasingly used in healthcare to monitor the quality of care from the patient's perspective. Relational PREMs gauge patients' experiences of their encounters with staff during treatment and functional PREMs measure their perceptions of more practical issues, such as the quality of clinic facilities. PREMs can be administered online and completed anonymously, and help clinics monitor the standard of care and take steps to improve care if indicated. An example of a relational PREM (the consultation and relational empathy measure) is shown in Figure 8.2.

Technology to Support New Users of MAR

In addition to "traditional" fertility patients – heterosexual infertile couples – new groups of people can now use MAR technologies to have children. These include cancer survivors, single women, lesbian and gay couples, transgender people, and women who freeze their eggs to avoid age-related infertility.

There is limited evidence about the particular needs of these new groups of MAR users, but it is important that clinic websites include relevant, high-quality, group-specific information about the treatment options available to them. Furthermore, administrative systems need to be adapted to each group's circumstances (e.g., a single woman should not be asked to provide the name of a partner), group-specific written

CARE Patient Feedback Measure for

Please write today's date here:

☐☐ / ☐☐ / ☐☐
D D   M M   Y Y

Please rate the following statements about today's consultation.

Please mark the box like this ✔ with a ball point pen. If you change your mind just cross out your old response and make your new choice. Please answer every statement.

How good was the practitioner at...	Poor	Fair	Good	Very Good	Excellent	Does not apply
1) **Making you feel at ease** (introducing him/herself, explaining his/her position, being friendly and warm towards you, treating you with respect; not cold or abrupt)	☐	☐	☐	☐	☐	☐
2) **Letting you tell your "story"** (giving you time to fully describe your condition in your own words; not interrupting, rushing or diverting you)	☐	☐	☐	☐	☐	☐
3) **Really listening** (paying close attention to what you were saying; not looking at the notes or computer as you were talking)	☐	☐	☐	☐	☐	☐
4) **Being interested in you as a whole person** (asking/knowing relevant details about your life, your situation; not treating you as "just a number")	☐	☐	☐	☐	☐	☐
5) **Fully understanding your concerns** (communicating that he/she had accurately understood your concerns and anxieties; not overlooking or dismissing anything)	☐	☐	☐	☐	☐	☐
6) **Showing care and compassion** (seeming genuinely concerned, connecting with you on a human level; not being indifferent or "detached")	☐	☐	☐	☐	☐	☐
7) **Being positive** (having a positive approach and a positive attitude; being honest but not negative about your problems)	☐	☐	☐	☐	☐	☐
8) **Explaining things clearly** (fully answering your questions; explaining clearly, giving you adequate information; not being vague)	☐	☐	☐	☐	☐	☐
9) **Helping you to take control** (exploring with you what you can do to improve you health yourself; encouraging rather than "lecturing" you)	☐	☐	☐	☐	☐	☐
10) **Making a plan of action with you** (discussing the options, involving you in decisions as much as you want to be involved; not ignoring your views)	☐	☐	☐	☐	☐	☐

Comments: If you would like to add further comments on this consultation, please do so here.

© CARE SW Mercer, Scottish Executive 2004: The CARE Measure was orginially developed by Dr Stewart Mercer and colleagues as part of a Health Service Research Fellowship funded by the Chief Scientist Office of the Scottish Executive (2000-2003).   4571132878

Figure 8.2 The CARE PREM

information should be available in printed and electronic downloadable formats, and staff should be trained to enquire about and strive to meet the unique needs of these groups.

Cancer Survivors

To preserve fertility potential (FP), people diagnosed with cancer in childhood or during their reproductive years can freeze reproductive material (gametes or ovarian or testicular tissue). However, to do this they need to be informed that this option is available. While studies indicate that cancer patients want and value information about FP options, there are many barriers for adequate oncofertility support, including lack of communication between cancer and fertility specialists[14,15]. Fertility clinics can support oncologists to discuss FP with their patients by providing information for health professionals on their websites and establishing a referral pathway that allows patients to be assessed by a fertility specialist and to access the FP option they choose with minimal delay to starting the cancer treatment they need.

Cancer patients want their future fertility addressed sensitively at the time of diagnosis and regard specialized websites and leaflets as the most helpful decision-support tools[16]. In their review of the availability and quality of information relating to female fertility in the context of cancer, de Man and colleagues[17] reported that fewer than half of fertility clinic websites included information about FP options. Hence, there is substantial scope for clinics to improve access to information about the impact of cancer treatment on fertility and the available FP options. The inclusion of a fertility-related decision aid may also help reduce decision regret[18]. Decision aids are used to help patients make decisions about complex health matters by providing information about the available options and their possible outcomes, and by clarifying personal values. They are designed to complement, rather than replace, discussions with health practitioners (see for example https://decisionaid.ohri.ca/).

Single Women

An increasing number of single women use MAR to become mothers. This is often a "plan B" for women who desire parenthood but have not found a partner who is willing to commit to parenthood. For some of these women it may be particularly painful to attend a service that caters predominantly for heterosexual couples. A content analysis of United States fertility clinic websites showed that, despite 90% of clinics accepting single women, less than one-third displayed explicit information about this on their website and only 10% displayed nondiscriminating statements[19]. Clinics that provide MAR for single women should endeavor to develop information that makes them feel included and respected and display this on their website in a section dedicated to single women.

Nonheterosexual People

Many LGBTQ individuals and couples who want children use MAR to achieve their parenthood goals. A review of fertility centers' websites showed that less than half included information relevant to LGBTQ couples and individuals[20]. Inclusion of material relevant to people with diverse gender identifications and sexualities on clinic websites is essential to ensure they can access inclusive information about the available MAR options.

Transgender youth contemplating medical gender reassignment can freeze gametes for future use if they wish. While Strang and colleagues found that most transgender youth were uninterested in using FP, they were open to the idea that fertility attitudes may change in adulthood[21]. This suggests that clinics should develop sensitively written information for this group about the option of freezing gametes and include this on their website.

FP for Nonmedical Reasons

As cryopreservation techniques have improved, the use of oocyte cryopreservation to protect against age-related infertility is increasing rapidly. Most women who freeze oocytes for nonmedical reasons do this because they lack a partner or have a partner who is ambivalent about parenthood[22,23]. To make informed decisions about FP, women need accurate information about the likelihood of a live birth; the cost of retrieval, storage, and later use of the eggs; and the possibility the eggs may remain unused. The ASRM cautions that "marketing this technology for the purpose of deferring childbearing may give women false hope and encourage women to delay childbearing." To avoid this, clinic websites should provide comprehensive and realistic information about all aspects of nonmedical oocyte cryopreservation.

Social Media, Online Support, and Digital Applications to Enhance the Patient Experience

In the last decade there has been increasing interest in studying the content and the effects of social media and digital interventions for people who experience fertility difficulties. A review of patient-focused interventions in reproductive medicine identified the following types of digital interventions: educational interventions, self-help interventions, human-supported therapeutic interventions, online support groups, and counseling services[24]. Common aims across interventions were information provision, support, and mental health promotion.

Social Media

In high-income countries, social media use is almost universal among people of reproductive age. Research indicates that using social media may be beneficial for information provision in the context of MAR care. In a survey of women attending a fertility clinic, most agreed that social media can enhance the patient experience. The most endorsed post topics were "education regarding infertility testing and treatment" and "myths and facts about infertility," which more than 90% of respondents expressed interest in. The least popular topic was "newborn pictures and birth announcements." Most clinic websites feature images of babies, but this finding suggests that patients might prefer alternative images.

Online Support

There are numerous online support groups for people experiencing fertility problems. Studies exploring the impact of participating in these report both benefits and disadvantages. Some evidence suggests that they can improve the relationship with the partner, reduce the sense of isolation, increase knowledge, and that they are perceived as

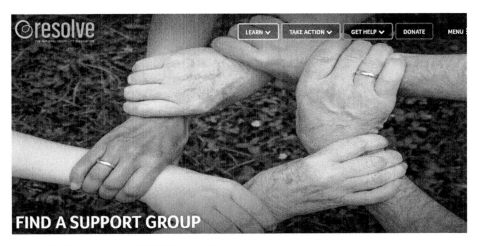

Figure 8.3 The home page of RESOLVE's website

a convenient way to receive and provide support anonymously. Downsides of online support groups include that reading stories about treatment failure may lead to over-whelming sadness and grief, and that use of online support can become obsessive. In a survey of more than 500 women and men attending fertility clinics in Canada, more than 80% expressed interest in online peer support. They stated preference for mobile accessibility, monitored peer-to-peer communication, and links to information. Higher levels of perceived stress were associated with greater interest in online support[25]. Figure 8.3 shows an image from the website of RESOLVE, the United-States-based national infertility association.

In their content analysis of infertility-related YouTube videos, Kelly-Hedrick and colleagues[26] identified two types of videos: personal and informational-educational videos. The most common content of the videos related to treatment outcomes, information sharing, emotional aspects of infertility, and advice to others.

Digital Applications

There is a growing number of mobile health tracking apps for chronic conditions, including infertility. However, few have been evaluated and little is known about if and how they benefit the user. Hence, there is a need for research to assess the effects of health apps, establish what makes an app user-friendly, and identify factors motivating users to continue to use the app[27].

When Technology Pulls Up Short And Human Interaction Is Preferred

While technology can enhance many aspects of communication in MAR care, there are times when patients prefer direct contact with clinic staff members. Comfortable, private spaces should be available for face-to-face staff–patient interactions. If staff communicate with patients by telephone, they need to ensure that the timing is convenient for the patient and that she or he has privacy during the conversation.

Discussing Treatment

In their review of studies examining patients' perspectives on fertility care, Dancet and colleagues[28] found that patients prefer to discuss treatment options and care with fertility staff. They also value the opportunity to discuss uptake or not of recommended treatment with staff and decisional support to deliberate their choice[1].

Most patients want test results explained in person, treatment information provided face-to-face, and in-person injection training. However, some prefer telephone consultations to discuss their treatment options and plans to reduce the number of visits to the clinic. Ideally, clinics offer patients their preference for discussing treatment options and plans. If they have urgent needs, patients want to be able to reach clinic staff via the telephone.

Delivering Bad News

In MAR, patients can receive several types of bad news throughout the treatment process (e.g., poor response to hormone stimulation, no oocytes retrieved, no fertilized oocytes, no embryos to transfer, no pregnancy, and pregnancy loss). After unsuccessful treatment, patients want fertility staff to offer additional psychosocial care and the opportunity to discuss the implications of ending treatment and concerns about the chance of a future pregnancy.

Delivering bad news requires that staff have well-developed communication skills and are mindful of how the news will affect the patient. As there are no specific guidelines for how to best manage difficult conversations in MAR, Leone and colleagues[29] suggest that using an adapted version of a six-step protocol for delivering bad news, which was developed for oncology care, can be helpful. It involves:

1. Preparing for the delivery of the bad news (find a private space, introduce oneself, involve significant others, sit down, manage interruptions)
2. Assessing the patient's perceptions of the situation
3. Assessing how much information the patient wants at the time and offering to be available and answering any questions as they may arise in the future
4. Providing information in small chunks and checking that the patient understands what is being conveyed
5. Responding compassionately to the patient's emotion and providing support
6. Summarizing the main points and discussing future hopes in terms of what is most meaningful to the patient and possible to achieve

Counseling and Emotional Support

While all fertility clinic staff should adhere to the evidence-based guidelines for patient-centered care and routinely provide psychosocial care to patients undergoing MAR treatment[1], there are times when individuals or couples need support from a mental health professional. This may relate to experiences of relationship problems, symptoms of depression or anxiety, repeated treatment failure, pregnancy loss, or other challenging circumstances.

Technology In Professional Education

The increasing complexity of MAR requires a highly specialized workforce. Patients want and expect fertility staff to be knowledgeable, trustworthy, empathetic, and supportive.

They value medical skills, respect, coordination, accessibility, information, comfort, support, partner involvement, and a good attitude of and relationship with fertility clinic staff[28]. To meet the needs of patients, all fertility clinic staff need comprehensive training in all aspects of MAR, including in communication. Technology offers excellent opportunities for fertility clinic staff to undertake basic and advanced training in the medical and psychological aspects of MAR through online distance education.

References

1. Gameiro S, et al. ESHRE Guideline: Routine Psychosocial Care in Infertility and Medically Assisted Reproduction – a Guide for Fertility Staff. *Hum Reprod*. 2015; 30(**11**): 2476–85.

2. Hammarberg K, et al. Quality of Information About Success Rates Provided on Assisted Reproductive Technology Clinic Websites in Australia and New Zealand. *ANZJOG*. 2018; 58(**3**): 330–4.

3. Wilkinson J, Vail A, Roberts SA. Direct-to-Consumer Advertising of Success Rates for Medically Assisted Reproduction: A Review of National Clinic Websites. *BMJ Open*. 2017; 7(**1**).

4. Harper J, et al. Adjuncts in the IVF laboratory: Where Is the Evidence for "Add-on" Interventions? *Hum Reprod*. 2017; 32(**3**): 485–91.

5. ASRM. The Role of Immunotherapy in In Vitro Fertilization: A Guideline. *Fertil Steril*. 2018; 110(**3**): 387–400.

6. Stephenson J, et al. Before the Beginning: Nutrition and Lifestyle in the Preconception Period and Its Importance for Future Health. *Lancet*. 2018; 391: 1830–41.

7. Ekstrand Ragnar M, et al. Development of an Evidence-Based Website on Preconception Health. *Upsal J Med Sci*. 2018; 123(**2**): 116–22.

8. Van Dijk MR, et al. Opportunities of mHealth in Preconception Care: Preferences and Experiences of Patients and Health Care Providers and Other Involved Professionals. *JMIR mHealth uHealth*, 2017; 5(**8**): e123.

9. Broughton DE, et al. Social Media in the REI Clinic: What Do Patients Want? *J Assist Reprod Genet*. 2018; 35(**7**): 1259–63.

10. Aarts JW, et al. Communication at an Online Infertility Expert Forum: Provider Responses to Patients' Emotional and Informational Cues. *J Psychosom Obstet Gynaecol*. 2015; 36(**2**): 66–74.

11. Haemmerli K, Znoj H, Berger T. Internet-Based Support for Infertile Patients: A Randomized Controlled Study. *J Behav Med*. 2010; 33(**2**): 135–46.

12. Cousineau, TM, et al. Online Psychoeducational Support for Infertile Women: A Randomized Controlled Trial. *Hum Reprod*. 2008; 23(**3**): 554–66.

13. Kingsley C, Patel S. Patient-Reported Outcome Measures and Patient-Reported Experience Measures. *BJA Education*. 2017; 17(**4**): 137–44.

14. Hammarberg K, et al. Cryopreservation of Reproductive Material Before Cancer Treatment: A Qualitative Study of Health Care Professionals' Views About Ways to Enhance Clinical Care. *BMC Health Serv Res*. 2017; 17(**1**): 343.

15. Logan S, et al. Clinician Provision of Oncofertility Support in Cancer Patients of a Reproductive Age: A Systematic Review. *Psycho-Oncology*. 2017; 27(**3**): 748–56.

16. Müller M, et al. Addressing Decisional Conflict About Fertility Preservation: Helping Young Female Cancer Survivors' Family Planning Decisions. *BMJ Sex Reprod Health*. 2018; 44(**3**): 175–80.

17. de Man AM, et al. Female Fertility in the Cancer Setting: Availability and Quality of Online Health Information. *Hum Fertil*. 2018; 1–9.

18. Peate M, et al. Making Hard Choices Easier: A Prospective, Multicentre Study to Assess the Efficacy of a Fertility-Related Decision Aid in Young Women with

Early-Stage Breast Cancer. *Br J Cancer*. 2012; 106(**6**): 1053–61.

19. Johnson KM. Excluding Lesbian and Single Women? An Analysis of U.S. Fertility Clinic Websites. *Women Stud Int Forum*. 2012; 35(**5**): 394–402.

20. Jin H, Dasgupta S. Disparities Between Online Assisted Reproduction Patient Education for Same-Sex and Heterosexual Couples. *Hum Reprod*. 2016; 31(**10**): 2280–4.

21. Strang JF, et al. Transgender Youth Fertility Attitudes Questionnaire: Measure Development in Nonautistic and Autistic Transgender Youth and Their Parents. *J Adolesc Health*. 2018; 62(**2**): 128–35.

22. Inhorn MC, et al. Elective Egg Freezing and Its Underlying Socio-Demography: A Binational Analysis with Global Implications. *Reprod Biol Endocrinol*. 2018; 16(**1**): 70.

23. Pritchard N, et al. Characteristics and Circumstances of Women in Australia Who Cryopreserved Their Oocytes for Non-Medical Indications. *J Reprod Infant Psychol*. 2017; 35(**2**): 108–18.

24. Aarts JW, et al. Patient-Focused Internet Interventions in Reproductive Medicine: A Scoping Review. *Hum Reprod Update*. 2012; 18(**2**): 211–27.

25. Grunberg PH, et al. Infertility Patients' Need and Preferences for Online Peer Support. *Reprod Biomed Soc Online*. 2018; 6: 80–9.

26. Kelly-Hedrick M, et al. "It's Totally Okay to Be Sad, but Never Lose Hope": Content Analysis of Infertility-Related Videos on YouTube in Relation to Viewer Preferences. *J Med Internet Res*. 2018; 20(**5**): e10199.

27. Birkhoff SD, Smeltzer SC. Perceptions of Smartphone User-Centered Mobile Health Tracking Apps Across Various Chronic Illness Populations: An Integrative Review. *J Nurs Scholarship*. 2017; 49(**4**): 371–8.

28. Dancet EAF, et al. The Patients' Perspective on Fertility Care: A Systematic Review. *Hum Reprod Update*. 2010; 16(**5**): 467–87.

29. Leone D, et al. Breaking Bad News in Assisted Reproductive Technology: A Proposal for Guidelines. *Reprod Health*. 2017; 14(**1**): 87.

The Economics of IVF: Evaluating the Necessity and Value of Public Funding

Evelyn Verbeke, Jeroen Luyten, and Thomas D'Hooghe

Overview of Public Funding of ARTs (In Selected Countries)

Infertility is recognized by the WHO as a condition leading to disability, and it is widely acknowledged that patients have a right to treatment[1]. One of the treatment options is ART. The International Glossary on Infertility and Fertility care defines procedures of ART as "all interventions that include the in vitro handling of both human oocytes and sperm or of embryos for the purpose of reproduction. This includes, but is not limited to, IVF and ET, ICSI, embryo biopsy, PGT, assisted hatching, gamete intrafallopian transfer, zygote intrafallopian transfer, gamete and embryo cryopreservation, semen, oocyte and embryo donation, and gestational carrier cycles. Thus, ART does not, and ART-only registries do not, include assisted insemination using sperm from either a woman's partner or sperm donor[2]." This right to treatment and the wide scope of ART that is available to patients is, however, confronted with limited and often already pressurized healthcare budgets. The unavoidable question is, therefore, which ART programs should be funded by public health insurance and which can be referred to private resources or private health insurance? This chapter discusses the public funding of ARTs and hence the access to them by large segments of the population.

Even though most common ARTs are technically available worldwide, substantial differences in access exist between and within countries (Figure 9.1). The most generous funding policies exist in Europe and the resulting highest utilization rates are found in Denmark, the Czech Republic, and Belgium. In Denmark 15 449 ART cycles per million females of reproductive age were performed, compared to 3844 cycles in Portugal. With a need for fertility treatments that is likely to be comparable over these countries, these large differences illustrate the impact of regulation and public funding on access to ARTs and hence the importance of finding a fair and sustainable funding scheme.

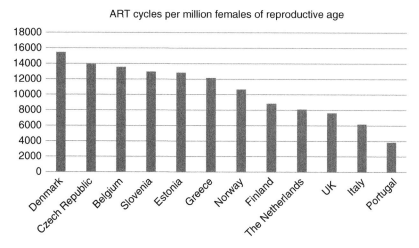

Figure 9.1 Data for 2014, for 12 European countries for which complete ART data are available. ART cycles include: IVF, ICSI, frozen-thawed ET (FER), egg donation, IVM, frozen oocyte replacement, and preimplantation genetic diagnosis (PGD) combined. For women aged 15–45 years.

Table 9.1 provides an overview of funding policies for the three most frequently used ARTs in Europe (in terms of treatment cycles in 2014): ICSI (46.6%), followed by FER (24.7%), and IVF (18.8%)[3]. Reported in this table are the European countries included in the International Federation of Fertility Societies (IFFS) and ESHRE reports and, to provide a broader comparison, six non-European countries (China, India, Israel, Japan, Russia, and the United States).

Ireland, Poland (since 2016), and Switzerland are the only European countries not providing any public coverage for ART programs. Of the countries that do offer reimbursement, all of them cover IVF. ICSI is not covered in the Czech Republic, Romania, and Slovakia. However, "complete coverage" does not imply that costs are fully reimbursed for *all* patients. Additional restrictions often apply: restrictions can be related to the patient's marital status, a maximum number of reimbursed cycles can be stated ranging from one cycle (Romania) to six (Belgium, Croatia, and Japan) and most countries impose an age limit for women, most commonly between 40 and 45 years. This age limit for reimbursement can differ from the legal age limit to undergo fertility treatment. In Belgium for example, the legal age limit for egg retrieval is 45 and 48 for ETs whereas these treatments are only reimbursed when the patient is younger than age 43 on the day of the insemination of the eggs[4].

These substantial discrepancies in public insurance coverage and usage of ART are the result of differences in priority setting and resource allocation among countries. How can policymakers decide which ART programs to fund, to which extent (fully or partially?), on which scale (for whom?) and how much money should in total be spent on ARTs? In this chapter, we explain some of the answers to these questions offered by cost-effectiveness analyses and their limitations in prescribing a fair and efficient public funding scheme.

Table 9.1 Overview of public health insurance coverage in selected countries

Country	Public coverage regulated by federal/national law[2]	Type of coverage provided[3]	Public insurance typically covers[2]				Age limit for coverage[2] (age women)
			IVF (maximum number of cycles)	ICSI	Cryopreservation of embryos for FP for medical indications	Cryopreservation of embryos from IVF cycle	
Austria	Yes	Partial (~70%)[4]	Yes	Yes	Yes	Yes	Yes (40, men 50)
Belarus	No	None	No	No	No	No	Yes
Belgium[5]	Yes	Complete	Yes (6)	Yes	No	Yes	Yes (43)
Bulgaria	Yes	Partial	Yes	Yes	No	Yes	Yes
China	No	None	No	No	No	No	NA
Czech republic[6]	Yes	Complete	Yes (4)	No	No	No	Yes (40)
Croatia[4]	NA	Partial	Yes (6)	NA	NA	NA	Yes (42)
Denmark	Yes	Complete	Yes	Yes	Yes	Yes	Yes
Estonia[4]	Yes	NA	Yes	Yes	No	Yes	Yes (40)
Finland	Yes	Partial	Yes	Yes	Yes	Yes	Yes
France[6]	Yes	Complete	Yes	Yes	Yes	Yes	Yes (43)
Germany[6]	Yes	Partial (50% + 25% federal states)	Yes	Yes	No	No	Yes (40, men 50)

Country							
Greece	NA	Partial	No	No	No	No	Yes (50 unrelated to reimbursement)
Hungary[4]	Yes	Partial (75%)	Yes (5)	Yes	No	Yes	Yes (45–49)
India	NA	None	No	No	No	No	NA
Ireland	No	None	No	No	No	No	No
Israel	Yes	Complete	Yes	Yes	Yes	Yes	Yes
Italy[6]	Yes	Partial (~65%)	Yes	Yes	No	Yes	Yes (50)
Japan	Yes	Partial	Yes (6)	Yes	No	Yes	Yes
Netherlands	Yes	Complete	Yes (3)	Yes	Yes	Yes	Yes (43)
Norway	Yes	Partial	Yes	Yes	Yes	Yes	No
Poland[6]	Yes	None	No	No	No	No	NA
Portugal[4]	Yes	Partial	Yes (3)	Yes	No	Yes	Yes (40)
Romania[6]	Yes	Partial (up to €1375)	Yes (1)	No	Yes	Yes	Yes (40)
Russia	Yes	Complete	Yes	Yes	No	No	No
Slovak Republic[4]	Yes	NA	Yes	No	No	No	Yes (40)
Spain[6]	No	Complete	Yes	Yes	Yes	Yes	Yes
Sweden[6]	Yes	Complete	Yes (3)	Yes	Yes	Yes	Yes (40, men 46)
Switzerland	NA	No	No	No	No	No	NA
Turkey	Yes	Partial	Yes	Yes	Yes	Yes	Yes

Table 9.1 (cont.)

Country	Public coverage regulated by federal/ national law[2]	Type of coverage provided[3]	Public insurance typically covers[2]					Age limit for coverage[2] (age women)
			IVF (maximum number of cycles)	ICSI	Cryopreservation of embryos for FP for medical indications	Cryopreservation of embryos from IVF cycle		
United Kingdom[6]	No	Partial	Yes (Scotland 3[7], Wales 2, Northern Ireland one 2-part cycle)	Yes	Yes	Yes		Yes (40)[1]
United States	No	No	No (6 – state specific)	NA	NA	No		NA

NA: not available
[1] Applicable in Scotland, Wales, and Northern Ireland; in England funding is region-dependent.

Health-economic Evaluation of ARTs

Available methods

Important first answers to the question which ART to fund are offered by economic evaluation studies. These analyses systematically compare two or more interventions on their costs and expected outcomes and express the value of the more promising option in terms of an incremental cost-effectiveness ratio (ICER): the additional costs required by a program per effect gained. Different types of economic evaluation exist, with the unit in which the health effects are expressed determining the type of evaluation. The broadest form of evaluation is cost–benefit analysis (CBA), expressing outcomes in monetary terms (e.g., the money equivalent of a clinical pregnancy achieved), which can be compared to the costs incurred. The advantage of this approach is that everything is expressed in money terms and this allows incorporating *all* possible sources of value of the outcome (not just clinical aspects of an ART but also its impact on, e.g., well-being to parents or economic benefits of having a child). The estimated return-on-investment can then be compared to the money returns of any other way of spending available resources. The disadvantage is that such a broad monetization of outcomes (especially of those that are typically kept out of the economic sphere) is considered ethically sensitive and highly challenging, and available estimates often lack reliability and validity.

Alternative evaluation techniques are cost-effectiveness analysis (CEA) and cost-utility analysis (CUA). In CEA, the outcomes considered are restricted to particular natural units of effects gained by the program. The ICER will hence be reported in terms of, e.g., a cost per live birth achieved, without specifying how valuable a live birth is. The advantage is its straightforwardness and, often, such estimates are meaningful to clinicians or decision-makers who have to allocate a ring-fenced budget (e.g., a fixed budget only to be used for ARTs). The disadvantage is that cost comparisons are only possible within the sphere of the particular effect that was considered (e.g., per live birth/per clinical pregnancy or per cycle) and a consensus on the most meaningful denominator for ARTs is currently lacking[5]. Furthermore, cost-effectiveness comparisons of interventions that operate in different healthcare domains, and where different health outcomes are "produced," become impossible. This means that from cost-effectiveness estimates we can judge which intervention is the most "technically efficient" one (producing desired outcomes at minimal cost), but we cannot judge whether the overall ART budget size is appropriate, and whether from a more global perspective on healthcare funding, resources are used where they create the most value (i.e., "allocative efficiency").

A third evaluation technique is somewhere in between CBA and CEA in terms of scope: CUA. Here, health effects are translated into "utilities" such as quality-adjusted life years (QALYs). A QALY is a generic "unit" of health, representing one life year in perfect health. Health effects of an intervention will thus consist of a certain number of QALYs gained, determined by the expected increase in life years, adjusted for the expected quality of life during those years. Quality-of-life weights are attributed to each year ranging from zero for a life that has the same value as death and one for a life in perfect health. CUA is the commonly-used method in the economic evaluation of healthcare programs as it allows cost-effectiveness comparisons of interventions in different health domains in terms of €/QALY, while avoiding the problems of monetizing health in CBA[6].

Cost-Effectiveness of IVF, ICSI, and Cryopreservation of Embryos

We summarize 18 recent cost-effectiveness studies in Table 9.2. This table is based on a targeted (rather than systematic) review, selecting recent economic evaluations related to the assessment of cost-effectiveness of IVF, ICSI, and cryopreservation of embryos (as these subjects were also included above). This search was conducted for articles published between 2009 and 2019, on PubMed and in high-impact journals focusing on fertility, human reproduction, or health economics. We discuss the reported cost-effectiveness results for the most common research questions and explore existing discrepancies in methodology.

Elective Single ET (eSET) Versus Double ET (DET)

The most common focus was the cost-effectiveness of elective single ET (eSET), compared to double ET (DET). Do the higher success rates of DET justify the higher risk of multiple gestation and related higher healthcare costs? In general, success rates of ART decline when women get older, leading to a lower risk of multiple gestation and hence higher cost-effectiveness of DET. Cost-effectiveness will consequently be dependent on the patient's age: according to Hernandez Torres and colleagues[7], eSET is not significantly more cost-effective for women younger than 38 years of age. However, Papaleo and colleagues[10] found eSET to be only cost-effective for women under 32 years. Roque and colleagues[11] reported 36 years of age as the age up to when eSET should be preferred. Fiddelers and colleagues[8] found eSET more cost-effective only for a willingness to pay (WTP) per program below €7350 [9] and reported eSET to be more cost-effective in general. As will be discussed later in the chapter, the public funding scheme will determine the patients' and clinics' behavior in choosing the most cost-effective option from their perspectives.

Freeze-Only Versus Fresh ETs

Freeze-all strategies in which all embryos are cryopreserved and transferred with delay are currently preferred for patients with high risk of OHSS, the need for preimplantation genetic diagnosis (PGD), preimplantation genetic screening, and impairment in endometrial receptivity owing to serum progesterone elevation during ovarian stimulation [10]. Improvements in cryopreservation techniques have shown freeze-all strategies to be an interesting alternative, as it has been proposed that the ET can be performed in a more favorable intrauterine environment, possibly improving ART outcomes, and hence increasing popularity of eSET compared to DET[11]. A freeze-all strategy may, however, also imply additional costs related to embryo cryopreservation, endometrial priming, extra medication use, and ultrasound scanning[12]. CEA provides the possibility of weighing these potentially higher success rates against the potential increase in costs.

Success rates of the freeze-all group were indeed found to be higher in a number of studies[10–12]. Papaleo and colleagues[10] also reported a lower average cost for the freeze-all group and hence found it to be more cost-effective. Roque and colleagues[11] reported a higher average cost per patient for the freeze-all strategy, but still identified freeze-all as the most cost-effective option because of the higher success rates.

Table 9.2 Summary of cost-effectiveness studies

First author (year) country of publication	Focus of study	No. of observations	Costs	Effectiveness	Reported cost-effectiveness (CE)
Elective single ET (eSET) versus double ET (DET)					
Crawford (2016) United States[1]	Assessment of costs and outcomes of DET and projection of the difference in costs and outcomes had the double ET cycles been performed as sequential eSETs	10 001 cycles DET, 4129 cycles eSET, patients <35 years with no prior ART use consisting of cryopreservation	*Average total cost per cycle, including infant-associated medical costs during first year of life:* $38 600 USD SET $58 100 USD DET (2006; USD)	*Cumulative birth rate* 68% SET 57.7% DET Multiple birth rates: 1.2% SET 24.7% DET	If 10 001 DETs would have been performed as sequential eSETs, this would have saved $195 million USD and increased live birth rates by 10.3% *(Own calculations:)* $56 765 USD per live birth SET $100 693 USD per live birth DET	Assumes no infants stillborn in a multiple birth, assumes same success rates for DET as the projected sequential eSET group. Ignores higher risk of drop-out in the case of eSET
Fiddelers (2009) The Netherlands[2]	The CE of seven different strategies is calculated. Three options are combined: 1. eSET in all patients 2. eSET in good-prognosis patients and DET in the remainder of patients (=STP)	308 couples who started their first IVF cycle	*Expected cost per couple per strategy:* 1. €16 381 2. €16 655 3. €17 092 4. €17 440 5. €16 999 6. €17 444 7. €18 046 (2003; €)	*Mean live birth rate per strategy:* 1. 39.6% 2. 43.3% 3. 43.3% 4. 45.7% 5. 47.5% 6. 49.9% 7. 53.4%	Combining several transfer policies was found not to be CE. The choice between eSET, STP and DET will be determined by the willingness to pay (WTP) <€7350: 3x eSET is to be preferred	Costs from societal perspective including health-care costs and costs outside healthcare sector. From two weeks before randomization up to six weeks after birth/two weeks after last ovum pickup

Table 9.2 (cont.)

First author (year) country of publication	Focus of study	No. of observations	Costs	Effectiveness	Reported cost-effectiveness (CE)	
	3. DET in all patients The seven strategies consist of: 1. Three eSET 2. eSET + two STP 3. eSET + STP + DET 4. eSET + two DET 5. Three STP 6. STP + two DET 7. Three DET				€7350 <WTP €15 250: 3x STP WTP >€15 250: 3x DET	
Hernandez Torres (2015) Spain[3]	CE of IVF-ICSI with eSET followed by the transfer of cryopreserved embryos (eSFET), versus DET	121 women <38 years old undergoing their first or second IVF cycle; 57 eSET + eSFET and 64 DET	*Average cost per patient:* €5641 eSET + eSFET €5562 DET (2012; €)	*Cumulative live birth:* 38.6% eSET + eSFET 42.19% DET group (differences were not statistically significant)	The chance of eSET + eSFET being CE is <50% for all threshold values *(ICER is not reported because no alternative was more effective for a higher cost)*	Costs include direct medical costs associated with AR treatment, pregnancy, childbirth, and neonatal care
Scotland (2011) UK[4]	Assessment of cumulative costs and consequences of eSET and DET in women commencing IVF	6153 women, 10 511 fresh cycles, 3106 frozen cycles. Up to three full cycles per patient	Not stated	Not stated	*Compared to eSET, DET leads to additional costs per live birth:* £27 356 age 32 £15 539 age 39	Time horizon of 20 years. In addition, use of QALYs to assess the cost-utility of the alternatives

			Cost/outcome	Birth rate	Cost per QALY / ICER	Notes
	with treatment ages 32, 36, and 39 years				*Additional cost per QALY of women for DET:* £28 300 age 32 £20 300 for age 39 =>eSET more CE for women ≤36 years old; older women: case-by-case decision	(Discount rate costs and effects: 3.5%) [2007; £]
Van Loendersloot (2017) The Netherlands[5]	CE of SET followed by an additional frozen-thawed (eSFET), compared to DET, in relation to female age	3390 patients undergoing IVF/ICSI	*Cost per strategy:* 1. SET + eSFET: €4491 for age 30 – €3623 for age 43. 2. DET: €5291 for age 30 – €3627 for age 43 (2010; €)	*Cumulative live birth rate:* 1. SET + eSFET: 36.8% at age 30 ≥49.7% at age 40. 2. DET: 34.1% at age 30 ≥11.7% at age 40	*ICER (DET compared to SET eSFET):* Age 30: €-29 032 Age 31: €-114 576 starting from age 32 DET becomes more cost-effective: Age 32: €50 348 ≥Age 43: €53 SET followed by eSFET is dominant over DET for women under 32 years. After the age of 32 DET was more effective but also more costly	Including direct medical costs, including cost of singleton/twin birth until six weeks after birth
Veleva (2009) Finland[6]	CE of eSET compared to DET	DET period (1995–1999): 1359 fresh embryo	*Total discounted costs per woman:* €4942 DET period €4584 eSET period	*Cumulative live birth rate:* eSET period: 41.7% DET period: 36.6%	€19 889 saved per term live birth in the eSET period:	Total treatment charges and medication costs for fresh and frozen

Table 9.2 (cont.)

First author (year) country of publication	Focus of study	No. of observations	Costs	Effectiveness	Reported cost-effectiveness (CE)
		cycles + 589 frozen cycles eSET period (2000–2004): 107 fresh and 683 frozen cycles	[2008; €], discount rate 3%		eSET with cryopreservation is more effective and less expensive than DET	embryo transfer (FET) cycles until pregnancy test. Costs from complications of ovarian stimulation were not included
Freeze-only versus fresh ETs					
Le (2018) Vietnam[7]	CE of freeze-only strategy compared to fresh ET after one complete IVF/ICSI cycle in women without PCOS	782 infertile couples	*Estimated total cost per couple:* €3906 freeze only €3512 fresh (2016; €)	*Live birth rate after one completed cycle:* Freeze only: 48.6% Fresh ET: 47.3%	*Estimated cost per live birth:* €8037/live birth for freeze-only strategy €7425/live birth for fresh ET strategy	Data from one single private IVF center in Vietnam. Costs include direct medical costs from randomization to delivery and treatment complications. Travel expenses and accommodation costs included

It should be noted that these costs are significantly lower compared to other studies |

Study	Description	Patients / Cycles	Mean cost per patient:	Cumulative live birth rate:	Mean cost per live birth:	Notes
Papaleo (2017) Italy[8]	CE of IVF freeze-all policy (entire cohort of embryos is cryopreserved) compared with fresh ET (only supernumerary embryos are cryopreserved)	Patients: 67 freeze-all policy, 189 fresh transfer	Mean cost per patient: Freeze-all: €6863 Fresh: €6952	Cumulative live birth rate: Freeze-all: 52.4% Fresh: 45.5%	Mean cost per live birth: Freeze-all: €13 101 Fresh: €15 279 =>Freeze-all more cost-effective although difference not significant	Only direct healthcare costs considered. Freeze-all patients: patients for OHSS risk, high progesterone levels on trigger day >1.5 ng/mL, detection of sacto, and hydrosalpinx and suspected endometrial pathology
Roque (2015) Brazil[9]	CE of freeze-all cycles compared to fresh ETs	530 ICSI cycles: 351 fresh embryo cycles and 179 freeze-all cycles	1. From perspective of private center policy and charges: Fresh: $7424 Freeze-all: $7598 2. Including cryopreservation and thawing costs from all patients in freeze-all group: Fresh: $7417 Freeze-all: $9020 (2015; USD)	Pregnancy rate (clinical pregnancy after confirmation of fetal heartbeat after 7–8 weeks of gestation) per cycle: 31.1% fresh group 39.7% freeze-all group	Total cost per ongoing pregnancy: Cost scenario 1 Fresh group: $23 060 Freeze-all group: $19 157 Cost scenario 2 Fresh group: $23 040 Freeze-all group: $22 742 Freeze-all policy is CE compared to fresh ET	Freeze-all patients: progesterone level on trigger day <1.5 ng/mL. Exclusion of patients with ovarian hyperstimulation syndrome (OHHS) risk. Exclusion of indirect costs

Table 9.2 (cont.)

First author (year) country of publication	Focus of study	No. of observations	Costs	Effectiveness	Reported cost-effectiveness (CE)
Delayed versus immediate IVF					
Eijkemans (2017) The Netherlands [10]	CE of immediate versus delayed IVF in relation to prognostic characteristics of the couple. Scenario one: wait one year and then undergo IVF for one year. Scenario two: immediate IVF during one year plus one year trying to conceive naturally	5962 couples with primary infertility	*Cost per scenario (two years):* *Unexplained infertility:* Scenario one: €6792 (age 30) to €6695 (age 38) Scenario two: €7379–€7331 *Endometriosis:* Scenario one: €6787–€6759 Scenario two: €6985–€7047 (2014; €)	*Live birth rate after scenario (= two years):* *Unexplained infertility:* Scenario one: 55% (age 30) to 33.8% (age 38) Scenario two: 55.1–37.6% *Endometriosis:* Scenario one: 43.5–24.6% Scenario two: 44.2–28.5%	*Discounted cost efficiency ratio (cost per live birth gained by immediate IVF):* *Unexplained infertility:* €56 500 (age 30) to €16 600 (age 38) *Endometriosis:* €19 400 (age 30) to €8700 (age 38) Recommendation for couples with unexplained infertility and female partner <31 years of age to wait three years before IVF can be considered	Excluding frozen embryos. Discount rate of 3.5% for costs and effects. Costs from societal perspective: direct and indirect medical and nonmedical costs (treatment, delivery and neonatal period)
Pham (2018) Australia[11]	CE of delaying IVF for six months in couples with unexplained infertility compared to immediate IVF treatment	8781 couples aged <40 years. 17 418 fresh and 10 230 frozen ET cycles	*Estimated out-of-pocket costs for three cycles IVF:* $7125–$19 500 AUS (assuming results are reported in AUS dollars; not stated)	*Live birth rate:* women <30 years: 64% women age 35–39: 48.7%	*Potential out-of-pocket savings if 90% of couples delayed IVF:* $4.7–$12.2 million AUS for 27 648 cycles (with total

Other studies

Groen (2013) The Netherlands [12]	CE of modified natural cycle (MNC) IVF or ICSI as an alternative for controlled ovarian hyperstimulation (COH) IVF or ICSI. Three scenarios: 1. Three cycles MNC versus one cycle COH with SET or (DET) + subsequent transfer of cryopreserved embryos 2. Six cycles MNC versus one cycle COH with strictly SET + subsequent transfer of cryopreserved embryos	1994 MNC cycles and 392 fresh COH cycles with subsequent transfer of cryopreserved embryos	Total costs per patient: MNC-IVF: €5415 MNC-ICSI: €5096 COH-IVF: €3221 COH-ICSI: €4167 (2009; €)	Cumulative live birth rate: MNC-IVF: 21.9% MNC-ICSI: 26.2% COH-IVF: 21.9% COH-ICSI: 32.1%	Costs per live birth: MNC-IVF: €24 728 MNC-ICSI: €19 452 COH-IVF: €14 710 COH-ICSI: €12 980 ≥COH dominates	Cost of singleton, twins included. Costs of medication, costs of treatment procedures, cost of ongoing pregnancies for singletons and twins including costs of pregnancy, delivery, and costs up to six weeks after delivery

Medicare cost savings up to $15.1 million AUS).

Delaying IVF for six months was found to substantially decrease costs without compromising live births

Table 9.2 (cont.)

First author (year) country of publication	Focus of study	No. of observations	Costs	Effectiveness	Reported cost-effectiveness (CE)
	3. Six cycles MNC with minimized medication (hCG ovulation trigger only) versus one cycle COH with SET or DET + subsequent transfer of cryopreserved embryos				
Messinger (2015) United States[13]	CE of TA to IVF in women who desire fertility after tubal ligation	2256 tubal anastomosis procedures, number of IVF observations not specified	Average cost not stated	*Ongoing pregnancy after TA:* Age <35: 63% Age 35–40: 44% Age >40: 5% *Ongoing pregnancy after IVF:* Age <35: 40% Age 35–40: 28% Age >40: 10% *Ongoing pregnancy after frozen IVF cycle:* Age <35: 39% Age 35–40: 35% Age >40: 21%	*Costs per ongoing pregnancy:* $16 466–$223 482 USD after TA $32 902–$111 679 USD for IVF => For women <40 years old, TA was found to be more CE; for women >41 years old IVF was the main CE approach The charges for IVF included physician visits, ultrasound and laboratory evaluation, oocyte retrieval, ICSI, ET, embryology fees, and all medications [2014; USD]

			Absolute costs per woman per scenario:	Cumulative live births:	ICER per scenario (€/additional live birth):	Costs of IVF cycle, ovarian reserve testing, and gonadotropin dose increase (limited cost inclusion)
Moolenaar (2011) The Netherlands [14]	CE of ovarian reserve testing in IVF. Scenarios: 1. No treatment 2. Up to three cycles of IVF limited to women <41 years old + no ovarian reserve testing 3. Up to three cycles of IVF with dose individualization of gonadotropins according to ovarian reserve 4. Up to three cycles of IVF with ovarian reserve testing and exclusion of expected poor responders after the first cycle	Computer-simulated cohort of subfertile women aged 20–45 years old, based on prospective cohort study following 4928 couples during 12 months	1. €0 2. €6917 3. €6678 4. €5892 (2008; €)	1. 9% 2. 54.8% 3. 70.6% 4. 51.9%	1. base case 2. €15 166 3. €10 837 4. €13 743 If society's WTP > €10 900, dose individualization according to ovarian reserve has the highest probability of being CE	
Tjon-Kon-Fat (2015) The Netherlands [15]	CE of: 1. IVF with ovarian stimulation, SET and subsequent cryocycles (three cycles) 2. IVF in an MNC (six cycles) 3. IUI-COH (controlled ovarian	602 couples with unexplained infertility, age 18–38	Mean costs per couple: €7187 for IVF-SET €8206 for IVF-MNC €5070 for IUI-COH (2013; €)	Live birth rate: IVF-SET: 52% IVF-MNC: 43% IUI-COH: 47%	ICER of IVF-SET compared with IUI-COH = €43 375 (IVF-MNC is more expensive and less effective> dominated). Both IVF strategies significantly more expensive than IUI-	ART treatment costs, medication, and pregnancy leading to delivery. Costs of pregnancy and delivery included

Table 9.2 (cont.)

First author (year) country of publication	Focus of study	No. of observations	Costs	Effectiveness	Reported cost-effectiveness (CE)
	hyperstimulation) (six cycles) as a first-line treatment for patients with unexplained subfertility				COH without being significantly more effective. CE of IVF-SET depends on society's WTP
Vitek (2013) United States[16]	CE of split IVF-ICSI for the treatment of couples with unexplained fertility	154 couples	*One cycle:* All IVF: $13 842 Split IVF-ICSI: $15 605 All ICSI: $15 605 *Two cycles:* All IVF: $21 197 Split IVF-ICSI: $22 176 All ICSI: $22 552 (2012; USD)	*Cumulative birth rates* *One cycle:* All IVF: 38.8% Split IVF-ICSI: 41.8% All ICSI: 41.8% *Two cycles:* All IVF: 61.6% Split IVF-ICSI: 64.9% All ICSI: 64.8%	Direct costs of IVF and ICSI (procedure, medication, and cryopreservation, ET, donor insemination) *ICER* *One cycle:* All IVF = base case (= preferred approach) Split IVF-ICSI: $58 766 USD All ICSI: $58 766 USD *Two cycles:* All IVF = base case Split IVF-ICSI: $29 666 USD (= preferred approach) All ICSI: $42 343 USD
Yilmaz (2017) Turkey[17]	Perinatal outcomes and CE of patients with advanced age. (Assessment of the current age cut-off in Turkey at 40 years old)	456 patients: 158 >39 years old,298 <39 years old	Mean cost per cycle for hormonal stimulation: ≥39 $1058 USD <39 $732 USD	*Clinical pregnancy rate:* ≥39 = 11.3% <39 = 38.6%	*Mean expense per pregnancy:* ≥39 = $9294 USD <39 = $1874 USD No cost details provided

1. Crawford S et al. Costs of Achieving Live Birth from Assisted Reproductive Technology: A Comparison of Sequential Single and Double Embryo Transfer Approaches. *Fertil Steril.* 2016; 105(**2**): 444–50.

2. Fiddelers AAA et al. Cost-Effectiveness of Seven IVF Strategies: Results of a Markov Decision-Analytic Model. *Hum. Reprod.* 2009; 24(**7**): 1648–55.

3. Hernandez Torres E et al. Economic Evaluation of Elective Single-Embryo Transfer with Subsequent Single Frozen Embryo Transfer in an in Vitro Fertilization/Intracytoplasmic Sperm Injection Program. *Fertil Steril.* 2015; 103(**3**): 699–706.

4. Scotland GS et al. Minimising Twins in in Vitro Fertilisation: A Modelling Study Assessing the Costs, Consequences and Cost-Utility of Elective Single Versus Double Embryo Transfer over a 20-Year Time Horizon. *BJOG.* 2011; 118(**9**): 1073–83.

5. van Loendersloot LL et al. Cost-Effectiveness of Single Versus Double Embryo Transfer in IVF in Relation to Female Age. *Eur J Obstet Gynecol Reprod Biol.* 2017; 214: 25–30.

6. Veleva Z, Karinen P, Tomas C, Tapanainen JS, Martikainen H Elective Single Embryo Transfer with Cryopreservation Improves the Outcome and Diminishes the Costs of IVF/ICSI. *Hum Reprod.* 2009; 24(**7**): 1632–9.

7. Le KD et al. A Cost-Effectiveness Analysis of Freeze-Only or Fresh Embryo Transfer in IVF of Non-PCOS Women. *Hum Reprod.* 2018; 33(**10**): 1907–14.

8. Papaleo E et al. A Direct Healthcare Cost Analysis of the Cryopreserved Versus Fresh Transfer Policy at the Blastocyst Stage. *RBM Online.* 2017; 34(**1**): 19–26.

9. Roque M, Valle M, Guimarães F, Sampaio M, Geber S Cost-Effectiveness of the Freeze-All Policy. *JBRA Assist Reprod.* 2015; 19(**3**): 125–30.

10. Eijkemans MJC et al. Cost-Effectiveness of "Immediate IVF" Versus "Delayed IVF": A Prospective Study. *Hum Reprod.* 2017; 32(**5**): 999–1008.

11. Pham CT, Karnon JD, Norman RJ, Mol BW Cost-Effectiveness Modelling of IVF in Couples with Unexplained Infertility. *RBM Online.* 2018; 37(**5**): 555–63.

12. Groen H, Tonch N, Simons AHM, van der Veen F, Hoek A, Land JA. Modified Natural Cycle Versus Controlled Ovarian Hyperstimulation IVF: A Cost-Effectiveness Evaluation of Three Simulated Treatment Scenarios. *Hum Reprod.* 2013; 28(**12**): 3236–46.

13. Messinger LB et al. Cost and Efficacy Comparison of in Vitro Fertilization and Tubal Anastomosis for Women After Tubal Ligation. *Fertil Steril.* 2015; 104(**1**): 32–8.e4.

14. Moolenaar LM et al. Cost Effectiveness of Ovarian Reserve Testing in Vitro Fertilization: A Markov Decision-Analytic Model. *Fertil Steril.* 2011; 96(**4**): 889–94.

15. Tjon-Kon-Fat RI et al. Is IVF – Served Two Different Ways – More Cost-Effective Than IUI with Controlled Ovarian Hyperstimulation? *Hum Reprod.* 2015; 30(**10**): 2331–9.

16. Vitek WS, Galárraga O, Klatsky PC, Robins JC, Carson SA, Blazar AS. Management of the First in Vitro Fertilization Cycle for Unexplained Infertility: A Cost-Effectiveness Analysis of Split in Vitro Fertilization-Intracytoplasmic Sperm Injection. *Fertil Steril.* 2013; 100(**5**): 1381–8.

17. Yilmaz N et al. Perinatal Outcomes and Cost-Effectivity of the Assisted Reproduction Pregnancies with Advanced Age: A Retrospective Analysis. *J Obstet Gynaecol.* 2017; 37(**4**): 450–3.

Apart from other study-specific factors, an important difference between studies is the observed population: Roque and colleagues[11] only considered patients with a progesterone level on trigger day >1.5 ng/mL. Papaleo and colleagues[10] also included patients for OHHS risk, detection of sacto- and hydrosalpinx, and suspected endometrial pathology. Because freeze-all strategies are not yet used for routine IVF treatments in all patient populations, broader evidence of "random patients" is still limited. Le and colleagues [12] evaluated cost-effectiveness based on one of the already available RCTs for women without PCOS. Success rates and costs for both strategies were similar for both randomized groups. Hence, the probability of freeze-all to be more cost-effective was found to be very low. In summary, a freeze-all strategy was found to be cost-effective for particular patient groups, but evidence of success rates, and hence cost-effectiveness, for more general groups is still very limited. Furthermore, a potential decrease in indirect costs of freeze-all because of lower maternal and perinatal morbidity was not considered in these studies, which may benefit the freeze-all case when considering cost-effectiveness in the long run[10].

Immediate Versus Delayed IVF

Temporarily postponing IVF may be cost-effective as natural conception may occur during this delay, naturally or by the use of cheaper, less-invasive techniques such as an improved diet or increased physical activity. The cost-effectiveness of delaying IVF depends on the type of infertility and the age of female patients (as success rates of young women decrease less rapidly). Pham and colleagues[13] reported a substantial decrease in out-of-pocket and Medicare costs by delaying IVF for six months for couples with unexplained infertility and a good prognosis for natural conception, while birth rates were minimally impacted. Eijkemans and colleagues[14] considered a delay of 12 months and concluded that couples with unexplained infertility and female partner younger than 31 should wait 3 years before considering IVF. For patients with endometriosis, however, the cost-effectiveness of delaying IVF was found to be low and only slightly dependent on the duration of fertility and female age.

Methodology Used in Reviewed CEAs

The types of costs considered, the time horizon in which costs and effects are measured, and the effectiveness measure used can all have an important impact on the study results. The available literature did not always account for the uncertainty regarding these issues. *Costs* were typically reported in terms of average cost per cycle or per patient (for the total number of cycles). The types of costs included are, however, very divergent and often not clearly specified. Costs considered in the selected articles included: direct medical costs associated with ART treatment, pregnancy, childbirth or neonatal care; travel expenses; and income lost due to visits. General guidelines determining which of these and other costs to include would facilitate direct comparisons of costs between different studies. The longest *time horizon* considered was six weeks after delivery[10,12,19], with the exception of Scotland and colleagues[17] who considered a time horizon of 20 years. This, in general, very limited time horizon may lead to suboptimal decision-making, as important long-term costs (borne by patients or the public health care system) are neglected. Also, all selected articles reported *effectiveness* in natural units and are hence to be labeled as CEAs. One study[18] reported the number of ongoing pregnancies, and others[11,19] the number of clinical pregnancies. All other studies reported outcomes in terms of live birth per cycle or cumulated live birth rate. Only Scotland and colleagues [17] considered health effects for the mother and expressed outcomes in terms of QALYs. For example a QALY loss was included when mothers had a disabled child or were infertile with the desire of having a child. The authors did not specify whether QALYs related to newborns were also taken into account[17]. Not including these QALYs, however, implies that a loss of quality of life of the newborn (for example related to prematurity or multiple gestation) would not be considered. This absence of information illustrates the vagueness of QALY usage in the context of ART, which we will discuss more extensively later in the chapter. A uniform effectiveness measure (the unit in which the ICER is reported) would facilitate comparisons between studies, but this requires consensus on the most meaningful denominator. In general, a cost per success (whether this is a live birth, clinical pregnancy, or ongoing pregnancy) is preferred, enabling the assessment of a completed program in terms of the desired outcome. Alternatively, evidence regarding the cost-effectiveness of one additional cycle could also be valuable. Taking into account decreasing marginal success rates (the success rate of every additional cycle will go down) might offer valuable information for policymakers when determining the maximum number of reimbursed cycles. However, evaluating a cost per cycle is ill-suited for the assessment of cryopreservation cycles (frozen ETs) as in this case only cumulative success rates provide meaningful information. A possible solution may be to calculate a cost per oocyte retrieval[5]. These last two alternatives may, however, both give rise to behavioral changes when competition among providers exists, which we will discuss later in the chapter.

Limitations of Cost-effectiveness Studies

Broader Costs and Benefits of ARTs

CEA was the dominant technique found to be used in evaluating ARTs. In general, cost-effectiveness studies only consider a limited variety of costs and effects and this for a limited period. To be able to assess the full value of ART – i.e., the value of an additional child – policymakers need to be aware of the much broader cost- and benefit-dimensions.

On the cost side, ART treatment leads to various *indirect costs* such as costs for psychological assistance or productivity loss during medical visits. These costs occur during, but also after, treatment and are often not included as analyses are generally performed from a more narrow payer perspective. Estimating productivity loss is difficult and can be country- and patient-dependent (according to the social security system and occupation of the parents). Moreover, should these costs be corrected for the fact that a newborn will him- or herself become a productive factor? Including these broader costs can hence lead to complex and incomparable evaluations. But, more fundamentally, ARTs can also give rise to *long-term costs* as significant medical, social, or educational costs might manifest related to, e.g., maternal complications, prematurity, twin births, or disability or other health problems of the newborn[20]. These costs occur throughout the life of mother and child, posing a significant burden on patients or society. For instance, there is some emerging evidence that ARTs in obese women lead to substantial and long-lasting complications in the newborn[21].

On the benefit side, commonly reported outcomes are "live birth" or "clinical pregnancy achieved." CEA evidence hence allows the ranking of alternative treatments, but does not provide an answer to how valuable a birth or pregnancy is and, hence, how much of the available budget should be spent on ARTs. Some have attempted to expand CEA to a CBA perspective by calculating a monetary value to society of an additional child based on proxies such as expected tax revenues. Connolly and colleagues calculated a lifetime discounted value of net taxes from an IVF-conceived child of £109 939 compared to £122 127 for a naturally conceived child[22]. A CBA perspective might appear specifically relevant for societies where population growth is below replacement level. However, taking into account the "expected societal revenues" of the newborn holds an important risk of discrimination. Calculating expected tax revenues would imply estimating the future educational or income level of the newborns, leading to a valuation of the potential newborn, which will most likely depend on the socioeconomic background of their parents. Alternatively, a parental WTP perspective can be applied: how much money are people willing to pay for a newborn child? Settumba and colleagues estimated the mean WTP of the general Australian population for one cycle of IVF to be $6135–$13 561 AUS (depending on the success rate of IVF)[23]. An Israeli study reported a WTP per cycle of $5482 for patients undergoing IVF and $4398 for the general public[24]. These values do not, however, reflect an objective valuation of a live birth as results will be influenced by various factors such as the perspective applied, the features of the survey, and the current national health insurance policy. Using a single monetary value for every live birth is hence a very abstract approach where significant amounts of information will be lost[23,24]. On the other hand, a live birth can also be translated into QALYs, but a consensus on how this can be done is lacking. Some authors argue that the use of QALYs is not appropriate as the conception of a new life cannot be considered an improvement of health[25,26]. If QALYs would be used to account for a healthy birth, ARTs would become extremely cost-effective compared to treatments in other health domains as it would produce a "lifetime" amount of QALYs for the newborn. The creation of QALYs per se would hence be considered a reason to bring someone into existence, leading to large investments in ARTs while neglecting the health of already existing people.

Lastly, although often forgotten in CEAs, undergoing ARTs influences the *well-being of the parents* substantially. Failure of treatments may have severe psychological consequences. Achieving a live birth can increase happiness, but having children may, however, again decrease life satisfaction in the long term[27]. In theory, these consequences can be included in CEA by using QALYs. Scotland and colleagues illustrated this approach by including maternal QALYs depending on the outcome of the ART treatment. (By contrast, the well-being of the partner was not considered.) Scotland and colleagues also illustrated the significant impact of a change in QALY weights on reported outcomes, however. This demonstrates the importance of a transparent and systematic use of QALYs, currently hampered by the lack of quality-of-life information related to infertility problems and ART[28,17]. Furthermore, the question also arises whether psychosocial consequences of fulfilling or not fulfilling the desire to have children can be captured sufficiently by the QALY approach[25].

Considering these much broader effects of ARTs raises the currently debated question whether ARTs fulfill a purely medical need (curing infertility) or a mere desire to have children and hence should or should not be covered by public health insurance [27,29]. Whereas this issue is fundamental to the question how to fund ART, it is in any case hard to argue that only purely clinical effects should be considered in funding decisions as health interventions always serve multiple purposes beyond generating health itself and, moreover, nonclinical problems (e.g., an unfulfilled wish to have a child) can lead to medical problems and associated costs more downstream (e.g., depression). Cost-effectiveness evidence unfortunately cannot provide an answer to these more fundamental questions, even when a method to systematically include broader costs and benefits is found.

A broader, related point that should be made in the context of evaluating ARTs and their broader costs and benefits is that what counts as a cost or benefit also depends on the underlying philosophical view on appropriate population size. Are more people better? We should be aware that cost-effectiveness studies of health interventions (especially CEA) are in general based on the ethical perspective of total utilitarianism, in which every live birth is perceived as a gain to society. In reality, this may not be the case, especially in countries with overpopulation. The field of population ethics provides interesting alternative perspectives based on what counts as an optimal population size. A discussion of these would, however, go beyond the scope of this chapter.

Behavioral Responses to ART Funding Schemes

A second aspect that is not considered in CEAs is the impact of behavioral responses as a result of changes in public funding. These unanticipated behavioral factors may, when not included, alter the assumptions underlying CEA and affect the resulting cost-effectiveness estimates.

Effects of price elasticity: Changes in public funding may give rise to changes in out-of-pocket costs and will, therefore, influence demand. When the patient's demand is *inelastic*, a percentage change in price leads to a smaller than 1% change in the number of treatments demanded. When demand is *elastic*, a percentage change in price gives rise to a larger change in demand. Chambers and colleagues estimated the price elasticity of ART-demand in developed countries and reported a relatively elastic demand when prices were in the midrange and a less elastic demand in the upper and lower price ranges. When out-of-pocket costs were considerably higher (e.g., in the United States), a small decrease in price did not have a significant impact on demand[20]. Decision-makers want to be aware of these possible changes in demand and their related economic consequences. For illustration, Connolly and colleagues estimated the change in IVF/ICSI demand after the change of German policy in 2004, introducing a 50% co-payment for patients. The short-term (12 months) price elasticity of demand after introducing patient payments of €1500–€2000 was estimated to be −0.36. (A 10% price increase results in a reduction of demand of 3.6%[30].)

Moral hazard and delayed IVF: Second, generous reimbursement of ARTs may encourage patients to undergo more ART cycles (even when expected success rates are limited) or to choose ART without first considering other less invasive methods. Van Loendersloot and colleagues[15] and Tjon-Kon-Fat and colleagues[16] illustrated the possible cost reductions by delaying IVF for young women with unexplained infertility without compromising expected live birth rates. Conversely, delaying ART for women with advanced age is not recommended as success rates more rapidly decrease. Higher age limits for women hence hold the risk that older women will also postpone treatment, leading to lower effectiveness of the reimbursed cycles[13,14,31].

Cross-border reproductive care: Existing national differences in regulation and public funding of ART gave rise to the increased use of cross-border reproductive care (CBRC), in which patients seek ART abroad. Slovakia is now the first country initiating public insurance coverage of CBRC[32]. The main reasons patients travel abroad for ART are lower costs, higher quality of treatments, or limited access to services in their home countries (e.g., because of income, sexual orientation, or advanced age). Popular countries for CBRC are the United States, Israel, Spain, Czech Republic, Denmark, and Belgium. Even though CBRC provides alternative opportunities to fulfill a child wish, it also holds some important risks. Firstly, CBRC is often facilitated by "brokers," connecting foreign patients online with local ART centers. Brokers may have other financial objectives, and language barriers hamper communication with local providers. The resulting asymmetrical information can lead to supplier-induced demand, encouraging unaware patients to undergo unnecessary or suboptimal treatments. For example DETs can be recommended to increase probability of a live birth without patients being aware of the risks and long-term consequences, which will be borne by the home country's health-care system. Furthermore, increased demand of foreign patients (with a higher WTP) may decrease local access for patients as they can be priced out of the market. Consequences of CBRC may therefore be substantial for patients and governments. Current CBRC regulation, however, is very limited and detailed information about the magnitude and scope of CBRC is lacking. Different international organizations such as the ESHRE and IFFS started data collection and are setting out general guidelines[33,34].

Patients maximizing success rates: Ultimately, a patient's objective will be to maximize the probability of a live birth while minimizing out-of-pocket costs. When ART is not fully funded by public health insurance, patients are likely to choose the program with the highest probability of a live birth, while limiting the number of cycles (and their related costs). For example in the United States, ART treatment costs are typically borne by patients, but pregnancy and infant-associated medical costs by health insurance. As a consequence, patients may be discouraged from choosing eSET compared to DET because they only consider the lower direct treatment cost of DET without the related medical "twin" costs borne by insurance[35]. Secondly, ART may be fully funded, but only for a limited number of cycles. This again encourages patients to increase their success rates per cycle without considering long-term consequences. Lastly, we also need to consider the fact that some patients might just prefer giving birth to twins. A Danish study (n=588, 2004) reported 58.7% of patients preferring twins[36]. A smaller but more recent American study (n=106, 2017) found that 61% of patients who never gave live birth preferred a singleton and 39% preferred twins[37].

Competition among clinics: Reported success rates are not only important for patients but also for providers when competition among ART clinics exists (e.g., in the context of CBRC). Reporting live birth rates per cycle encourages clinics to improve their reputation by increasing the number of DETs, disregarding the conclusions of cost-effectiveness studies we previously discussed. Attention on this problem has increased and eSET is now encouraged by raising awareness of patients and by adaptations of ART funding policies[38]. For example a higher uptake of eSET was found to be closely related to more generous ART funding schemes[39]. Countries can also specify the number of embryos allowed during ET to obtain reimbursement. Belgium was the first country to link reimbursement of laboratory costs to transfer of a restricted number of embryos (dependent on female age and rank of cycle) to reduce the risk of multiple gestation.

Table 9.3 Legal access to IVF or ART services based on sexual orientation (IFFS, 2016)

Country	Stable heterosexual relationship required	Access for single women	Access for single men	Access for female same-sex couples	Access for male same-sex couples
Austria	Yes	NA	NA	NA	NA
Belarus	No	Yes	No	NA	NA
Belgium	No	Yes	Yes	Yes	Yes
Bulgaria	No	Yes	No	Yes	No
China	Yes	NA	NA	NA	NA
Czech Republic	Yes	NA	NA	NA	NA
Croatia	NA	NA	NA	NA	NA
Denmark	No	Yes	No	Yes	No
Estonia	No	Yes	No	Yes	No
Finland	No	Yes	Yes	Yes	Yes
France	Yes	NA	NA	NA	NA
Germany	No	Yes	No	Yes	No
Greece	No	Yes	No	No	No
Hungary	Yes	NA	NA	NA	NA
India	NA	NA	NA	NA	NA
Ireland	No	Yes	No	Yes	Yes
Israel	No	Yes	NA	No	No
Italy	Yes	NA	NA	NA	NA
Japan	Yes	NA	NA	NA	NA
Netherlands	No	Yes	NA	Yes	NA
Norway	Yes	NA	NA	NA	NA
Poland	NA	NA	NA	NA	NA
Portugal	Yes	NA	NA	NA	NA
Romania	No	Yes	No	No	No
Russia	No	Yes	No	NA	No
Slovak Republic	Yes	NA	NA	NA	NA
Spain	No	Yes	NA	Yes	No
Sweden	Yes	NA	NA	NA	NA
Switzerland	Yes	NA	NA	NA	NA
Turkey	Yes	NA	NA	NA	NA

Table 9.3 (cont.)

Country	Stable heterosexual relationship required	Access for single women	Access for single men	Access for female same-sex couples	Access for male same-sex couples
United Kingdom	No	Yes	Yes	Yes	Yes
United States	No	Yes	Yes	Yes	Yes

NA: no answer was stated

Furthermore, a maximum number of six fresh cycles was determined, not including cryopreservation cycles, and therefore encouraging additional frozen ETs[4]. Peeraer and colleagues demonstrated a 50% reduction in multiple pregnancy rates as a result of this policy implementation, without a negative impact on the cumulative delivery rate of patients[40]. As a consequence, in this context, calculating the cost per oocyte retrieval seems the most meaningful cost-effectiveness measure. But this again holds a risk as it may encourage more aggressive ovarian stimulation when the number of oocyte retrievals is limited[5]. This risk needs to be managed taking into account the risk of OHSS by balancing the intensity of ovarian stimulation (gonadotrophin dosing), by the choice of ovulation triggering (GnRH agonist when OHSS risk is high), and the option of freezing all retrieved oocytes/embryos.

Equity

Last, CEAs do not consider distributional effects of public funding schemes. General global access to ART is increasing, but barriers to utilization still exist. Summarized below are three grounds on which ART funding can lead to the exclusion of specific patient groups and consequently to unequal, and potentially inequitable, access.

Socioeconomic status: First, access to ART will depend on the socioeconomic status of a patient. Access to financial means will determine whether the patient can pay out-of-pocket costs of publicly funded programs or supplementary treatments in private clinics. Additionally, access is determined by indirect factors such as access to information, flexibility at work, and support from families and friends. Furthermore, the risk of infertility and hence the demand for ART is also related to socioeconomic status, as it is determined by the work and living environment of patients and behavioral factors such as smoking, drug use, or obesity.

Cultural differences: Second, cultural differences exist with regard to the perceived optimal family size and hence the importance of fertility. For example in developing countries, demand for ART is most prevalent as infertility or childlessness causes a severe burden on individuals. Paradoxically, access in these countries is very limited as priority is given to other health domains[41]. The question arises of whether parents should be given equal opportunity to fulfill their child wish, or to achieve their desired family size. In the first case, we can argue that achieving one healthy birth is sufficient to fulfill this wish and public funding can be limited to cases of primary infertility. Limiting the number of children a couple can have when seeking ART treatment seems reasonable, considering the limited health-care budget. On the other hand, it will be difficult to justify a universal limit that will allow some cultural groups to achieve their desired family size and others not.

Sexual orientation: Last, barriers to utilization of ART based on the sexual orientation of patients are not uncommon (Table 9.3)[32]. When patients do not have access to treatment, they will have to turn to (often more expensive) private providers or CBRC. In 13 of the 32 selected countries, a stable heterosexual relationship is required. Discrimination based on sexual orientation might result from the idea that patients should only be provided the opportunity of achieving "normal functioning." Even when same-sex couples are fertile, achieving a live birth is just not part of their normal functioning. On the other hand, one might consider same-sex couples and single parents more eligible for reimbursement because they suffer the injustice of not being able to achieve the same family goals heterosexual couples might have[27].

Conclusion

Differences in national health insurance coverage of ARTs give rise to significant variations in utilization rates between countries, illustrating the importance of a well-conceived funding scheme. This chapter discussed the challenges of setting out an optimal and justifiable public funding scheme for ARTs.

Economic evaluation evidence allows the ranking of alternative treatments based on their value for money, with value defined in either more narrow or broader terms. We summarized evidence of recent cost-effectiveness studies on ARTs. When interpreting outcomes, however, we need to be aware of the differences between studies in terms of costs and time horizon considered and effectiveness measure used. Reaching consensus on a uniform denominator for cost-effectiveness studies of ARTs is not straightforward as broader consequences and the local policy framework need to be taken into account.

The narrow perspective of CEA has, nevertheless, some important limitations in prescribing funding. Firstly, policymakers need to consider the broader social value of ARTs and the broader range of relevant costs that can emerge. However, considering broader costs and benefits raises the question where to draw the line and how to determine to which extent ARTs fulfill a purely medical need or whether their goals are broader. This is important to determine as the answer here will affect which type of (broad or narrow) evaluation framework is most appropriate to prescribe public funding. Second, CEAs neglect behavioral reactions and the consequences of patients and providers trying to optimize their own outcomes and not choosing the most cost-effective alternative from a societal perspective. Last, how can equal access be provided without discriminating against groups based on socioeconomic status, cultural differences, or sexual orientation?

Including these broader dimensions in the evaluation of ARTs and in subsequent priority-setting choices poses a major challenge for policymakers. A systematic and transparent method is needed to enable more consistent and uniform decision-making regarding resource allocation for ARTs not only on a micro level to determine which particular ART programs should be funded and to which extent but also on a macro level to determine the scope of public resources that should go to ARTs as a whole.

References

1. WHO. Infertility Definitions and Terminology. Online article. http://www.who.int/reproductivehealth/topics/infertility/definitions/en/

2. Zegers-Hochschild F et al. The International Glossary on Infertility and Fertility Care, 2017. *Hum Reprod.* 2017; 32 (**9**): 1786–801.

3. De Geyter C et al. ART in Europe, 2014: Results Generated from European Registries by ESHRE. The European IVF-monitoring Consortium (EIM) for the European Society of Human Reproduction and Embryology (ESHRE). *Hum Reprod.* 2018; 33(**9**): 1586–601.

4. Centrum voor Reproductieve Geneeskunde. Information About the Cost of an Assisted Reproductive Treatment for Belgian Patients. Universitair Ziekenhuis Brussel. 2016.

5. Martins WP, Niederberger C, Nastri CO, Racowsky C. Making Evidence-Based Decisions in Reproductive Medicine. *Fertil Steril.* 2018; 110(**7**): 1227–30.

6. Drummond MF, Sculpher MJ, Torrance GW, O'Brien BJ, Stoddart GL. *Methods for the Economic Evaluation of Health Care Programmes* (3rd Edition). Great Britain: Oxford University Press; 2005.

7. Hernandez Torres E et al. Economic Evaluation of Elective Single-Embryo Transfer with Subsequent Single Frozen Embryo Transfer in an in Vitro Fertilization/Intracytoplasmic Sperm Injection Program. *Fertil Steril.* 2015; 103 (**3**): 699–706.

8. Fiddelers AAA et al. Cost-Effectiveness of Seven IVF Strategies: Results of a Markov Decision-Analytic Model. *Hum Reprod.* 2009; 24(**7**): 1648–55.

9. Veleva Z, Karinen P, Tomas C, Tapanainen JS, Martikainen H. Elective Single Embryo Transfer with Cryopreservation Improves the Outcome and Diminishes the Costs of IVF/ICSI. *Hum Reprod.* 2009; 24(**7**): 1632–9.

10. Papaleo E et al. A Direct Healthcare Cost Analysis of the Cryopreserved Versus Fresh Transfer Policy at the Blastocyst Stage. *Reprod Biomed Online.* 2017; 34(**1**): 19–26.

11. Roque M, Valle M, Guimarães F, Sampaio M, Geber S. Cost-Effectiveness of the Freeze-All Policy. *JBRA Assist Reprod.* 2015; 19(**3**): 125–30.

12. Le KD et al. A Cost-Effectiveness Analysis of Freeze-Only or Fresh Embryo Transfer in IVF of Non-PCOS Women. *Hum Reprod.* 2018; 33(**10**): 1907–14.

13. Pham CT, Karnon JD, Norman RJ, Mol BW. Cost-Effectiveness Modelling of IVF in Couples with Unexplained Infertility. *Reprod Biomed Online.* 2018; 37 (**5**): 555–63.

14. Eijkemans MJC et al. Cost-Effectiveness of "Immediate IVF" Versus "Delayed IVF": A Prospective Study. *Hum Reprod.* 2017; 32(**5**): 999–1008.

15. van Loendersloot LL et al. Cost-Effectiveness of Single Versus Double Embryo Transfer in IVF in Relation to Female Age. *Eur J Obstet Gynecol Reprod Biol.* 2017; 214: 25–30.

16. Tjon-Kon-Fat RI et al. Is IVF – Served Two Different Ways – More Cost-Effective Than IUI with Controlled Ovarian Hyperstimulation? *Hum Reprod.* 2015; 30 (**10**): 2331–9.

17. Scotland GS et al. Minimising Twins in In Vitro Fertilisation: A Modelling Study Assessing the Costs, Consequences and Cost-Utility of Elective Single Versus Double Embryo Transfer over a 20-Year Time Horizon. *BJOG.* 2011; 118(**9**): 1073–83.

18. Messinger LB et al. Cost and Efficacy Comparison of in Vitro Fertilization and Tubal Anastomosis for Women After Tubal Ligation. *Fertil Steril.* 2015; 104(**1**): 32–8.e4.

19. Yilmaz N et al. Perinatal Outcomes and Cost-Effectivity of the Assisted Reproduction Pregnancies with Advanced Age: A Retrospective Analysis. *J Obstet Gynaecol.* 2017; 37(**4**): 450–3.

20. Chambers GM, Sullivan EA, Ishihara O, Chapman MG, Adamson GD. The Economic Impact of Assisted Reproductive Technology: A Review of Selected Developed Countries. *Fertil Steril.* 2009; 91(**6**): 2281–94.

21. Williams CB, Mackenzie KC, Gahagan S The Effect of Maternal Obesity on the Offspring. *Clin Obstet Gynecol.* 2014; 57 (**3**): 508–15.

22. Connolly M, Gallo F, Hoorens S, Ledger W. Assessing Long-Run Economic Benefits Attributed to an IVF-Conceived Singleton Based on Projected Lifetime Net Tax Contributions in the UK. *Hum Reprod.* 2008; 24(**3**): 626–32.

23. Settumba SN, Shanahan M, Botha W, Ramli MZ, Chambers GM. Reliability and Validity of the Contingent Valuation Method for Estimating Willingness to Pay: A Case of In Vitro Fertilisation. *Appl Health Econ Health Policy.* 2018.

24. Spiegel U, Gonen LD, Templeman J. Economic Implications of in Vitro Fertilization Using Willingness to Pay. *J Public Health.* 2013; 21(**6**): 535–57.

25. Devlin N, Parkin D. Funding Fertility: Issues in the Allocation and Distribution of Resources to Assisted Reproduction Technologies. *Hum Fertil (Camb).* 2003; 6 (**1**): S2–6.

26. Collins JA. An International Survey of the Health Economics of IVF and ICSI. *Hum Reprod Update.* 2002; 8(**3**): 265–77.

27. McTernan E. Should Fertility Treatment be State Funded? *J Appl Philos.* 2015; 32 (**3**): 227–40.

28. Hubens K, Arons AMM, Krol M. Measurement and Evaluation of Quality of Life and Well-Being in Individuals Having or Having Had Fertility Problems: A Systematic Review. *Eur J Contracep Reprod Health Care.* 2018; 1–10.

29. McMillan J. Allocating Fertility Services by Medical Need. *Hum Fertil.* 2001; 4(**1**): 11–13.

30. Connolly MP, Griesinger G, Ledger W, Postma MJ. The Impact of Introducing Patient Co-Payments in Germany on the Use of IVF and ICSI: A Price-Elasticity of Demand Assessment. *Hum Reprod.* 2009; 24(**11**): 2796–800.

31. Dolan P, Rudisill C. Babies in Waiting: Why Increasing the IVF Age Cut-off Might Lead to Fewer Wanted Pregnancies in the Presence of Procrastination. *Health Policy.* 2015; 119(**2**): 174–9.

32. IFFS Surveillance 2016. Global Reproductive Health. Online article. https://journals.lww.com/grh/Fulltext/2016/09000/IFFS_Surveillance_2016.1.aspx

33. Salama M. Cross Border Reproductive Care (CBRC): A Growing Global Phenomenon with Multidimensional Implications (a Systematic and Critical Review). *J Assist Reprod Genet.* 2018; 35 (**7**): 1277–88.

34. Präg P, Mills MC Assisted Reproductive Technology in Europe: Usage and Regulation in the Context of Cross-Border Reproductive Care. In: Kreyenfeld M, Konietzka D (eds.) *Childlessness in Europe: Contexts, Causes, and Consequences.* Cham: Springer International Publishing; 2017: 289–309.

35. Crawford S et al. Costs of Achieving Live Birth from Assisted Reproductive Technology: A Comparison of Sequential Single and Double Embryo Transfer Approaches. *Fertil Steril.* 2016; 105(**2**): 444–50.

36. Højgaard A, Ottosen LDM, Kesmodel U, Ingerslev HJ. Patient Attitudes Towards Twin Pregnancies and Single Embryo Transfer – a Questionnaire Study. *Hum Reprod.* 2007; 22(**10**): 2673–8.

37. Libby V, Thakore S, Weinerman R, Goldfarb J. Change in Patient Attitude Towards Multiple Gestation Pregnancies and Selective Fetal Reduction over 20 Years. *Fertil Steril.* 2018; 109(**3**): e36.

38. Multiple Pregnancies Following Assisted Conception. *BJOG.* 2018; 125(**5**): e12–18.

39. Maheshwari A, Griffiths S, Bhattacharya S. Global Variations in the Uptake of Single Embryo Transfer. *Hum Reprod Update.* 2011; 17(**1**): 107–20.

40. Peeraer K et al. The Impact of Legally Restricted Embryo Transfer and Reimbursement Policy on Cumulative Delivery Rate After Treatment with Assisted Reproduction Technology. *Hum Reprod.* 2014; 29(**2**): 267–75.

41. Ombelet W. Is Global Access to Infertility Care Realistic? The Walking Egg Project. *Reprod Biomed Online.* 2014; 28(**3**): 267–72.

<table>
<tr><td>**Chapter**

10</td><td># Medical and Elective Fertility Preservation: Options and Suggestions for a Patient-Centered Approach

Pasquale Patrizio and Marcia Inhorn</td></tr>
</table>

Introduction

Fertility preservation (FP) has become a specialized branch of reproductive medicine aimed at preserving the potential for future genetic parenthood for young adults, or even children, at risk of sterility before undergoing cancer treatment. Thanks to more refined chemotherapy and radiotherapy protocols, the five-year survival rates for many cancers have steadily increased; e.g., survivorship for Hodgkin's lymphoma went from 86% to 98% and for breast cancer from 78% to 91% in the last 25 years[1,2]. However, the risk of sterilization or early menopause by the effects of ionizing radiation or alkylating agents such as cyclophosphamide, procarbazine, and platinum-based drugs is high and therefore preserving future fertility is of paramount importance for the future quality of life-adjusted years[3,4].

Lately, the indications for FP have expanded and today an increasing number of healthy, mostly single and unpartnered, women are also resorting to FP, namely elective oocyte cryopreservation, to safeguard their wishes of future reproduction while postponing motherhood[5,6]. All the options available for FP are considered established and standard of care, except ovarian tissue cryopreservation and re-transplantation that is still considered experimental (although the ASRM at the time of writing is evaluating whether to remove the label of experimental). In this chapter we describe the various options available to preserve fertility in women for medical and nonmedical indications and will elucidate the ideal, patient-centered approach for medical and elective oocyte cryopreservation as revealed by some recent studies[7,8].

Medical Indications and Options for FP

International guidelines on FP in patients with cancer strongly suggest that all patients of reproductive age at risk of iatrogenic infertility should be referred to reproductive specialists prior to starting potentially gonadotoxic treatments, so as to be fully informed about FP options[4,9]. Ovarian dysfunction after chemotherapy has been well described. The nature and extent of this damage depends on the type of the chemotherapy drug given, the dose received, the underlying health conditions, and the age of the patient at the time of treatment. For example, cytotoxic agents (cyclophosphamide and procarbazine) are considered particularly gonadotoxic, able to deplete the primordial ovarian follicular pool and thus at high risk for causing premature ovarian insufficiency (POI). Women receiving preconditioning and radiotherapy for bone marrow transplantation are also at a high risk for future infertility[4,9]. Although Wallace and colleagues[10] developed an age-predictive model for ovarian failure after treatment with a known dose of radiotherapy, because of the varied and individual nature of the gonadal insult after radiotherapy, it is often extremely difficult to give a young patient an accurate assessment of the risk to fertility and the likelihood of POI after cancer treatment. Given the inability to predict future fertility, whenever possible, it is always better to offer potential benefits of cryopreservation.

An increasing number of patients diagnosed with non-oncological conditions are also being referred to specialists for discussing FP[4]. These are patients with autoimmune diseases (systemic lupus erythematosus, Behcet's disease, granulomatosis with polyangiitis (formerly known as Wegener's granulomatosis), and so on), or requiring hematopoietic stem cell transplantation (autologous or allogeneic) (sickle cell anemia, thalassemia major, aplastic anemia), or at risk of POI for known genetic causes (e.g., mosaic Turner syndrome, galactosemia), or transgender.

A number of options are available for FP and the most commonly offered are: (a) oocyte freezing, (b) embryo freezing, (c) ovarian transposition, (d) suppression of folliculogenesis, and (e) ovarian tissue cryopreservation. Some of these options are compared in Table 10.1.

Oocyte and embryo cryopreservation via IVF are the most widely established and available treatment options for both preservation and postponement of fertility[4,9]. In general, the IVF procedure requires, at the most, two weeks of delaying treatment and involves stimulation of the patient's ovaries with specific protocols, which can be started at any point in the menstrual cycle (random starts). For patients with diagnosis of breast cancer, letrozole (an aromatase inhibitor) is part of the protocol to keep the levels of E2 low. Oocyte retrieval is carried out via ultrasound-guided transvaginal aspiration and metaphase II oocytes are either cryopreserved by vitrification or, in the event of embryo freezing, they are fertilized, and the resulting embryos cryopreserved on day one as two pronuclei, or about five days later at the blastocyst stage of development. When the patient is cancer free and cleared to attempt pregnancy, in the event of POI, she can use the oocytes or the cryopreserved embryos for a chance at motherhood.

Transposition of the ovaries (oophoropexy) outside of the pelvis is indicated in patients who require pelvic radiation. This conservative surgical option may be preferred in either prepubertal patients or patients who hope to maintain long-term endocrine function. The procedure is performed by laparoscopy[11] and has been successful in 16–90% of the reported cases, with the variation likely a result of the inability to prevent scatter radiation, differing doses of radiation used, and the use of combination chemotherapy. It is important to note that oophoropexy must be performed close to the time of radiotherapy as the ovaries may migrate over extended periods back into the pelvis. Also,

Table 10.1 Comparison of methods of FP

	Oocyte cryopreservation	Embryo cryopreservation	Ovarian tissue cryopreservation	Suppression of folliculogenesis
Requires ovarian stimulation	Yes	Yes	No	No
Need partner or donor sperm	No	Yes	No	No
Treatment delay (two weeks)	Yes	Yes	No	No
Requires surgery	No	No	Yes	No
Applicable in prepubertal girls	No	No	Yes	No
Return endocrine function	No	No	Yes	Yes/no
Live births	Yes	Yes	Yes	Yes
Experimental	No	No	Yes	Unclear

patients should be aware that once cured from their cancer, due to the new location of the ovaries away from the fallopian tubes, to achieve a pregnancy they may require IVF.

Suppression of folliculogenesis with GnRHa for FP is still controversial with conflicting results about the efficacy in protecting from the risk of POI to the point that the American Society of Clinical Oncology[12] still suggest oocyte or embryo freezing if the cancer treatment can be delayed for two weeks (Table 10.1 provides a comparison of methods for FP).

When the time interval between cancer diagnosis and initiation of treatment is sufficient and patients choose to undergo COS for oocyte retrieval (medical egg freezing), they should be counseled that, in general, conventional COS can provide an average of 8.5 ± 6.4 metaphase II (MII) oocytes for vitrification per cycle, depending on the woman's age and ovarian reservation[13]. However, patients should also be made aware that, so far, only very few women with cancer have returned to use their cryopreserved oocytes; therefore, the future success rate quoted is mainly based on data from egg donation cases and from nonmedical cases of oocyte cryopreservation. Extrapolating from these cases, it is suggested that around 20 vitrified oocytes are required to achieve a live birth[14,15].

Ovarian tissue cryopreservation (OTC) is the only possible option if the chemotherapy or radiotherapy must start immediately, with no time for ovarian stimulation. Although the life span of re-transplanted ovarian tissue varies, reports of continuation of function of re-transplanted frozen/thawed ovarian cortical strip for more than 5–10 years, and close to 100 healthy live births, have been documented[16].

OTC has not been reserved solely for women with malignant disease. Hematopoietic stem cell transplantation (HSCT) has been increasingly used in recent decades for noncancerous disease such as benign hematological disease (sickle cell anemia, thalassemia major, and aplastic anemia) and autoimmune disease previously unresponsive to immunosuppressive therapy (systemic lupus erythematosus, Behcet's disease, granulomatosis with polyangiitis, and autoimmune thrombocytopenia)[17]. A large retrospective survey of pregnancy outcomes after HSCT involving 37 362 patients revealed that only 0.6% of patients conceived after autologous or allogenic HSCT. Other benign diseases have high risk of POI such as recurrent large ovarian endometriomas or recurrent ovarian mucinous cysts, and mosaic Turner syndromes[18].

For prepubertal girls, isolation and cryopreservation of ovarian cortical strips/primordial follicles followed by future re-transplant or in vitro maturation of gametes when fertility is desired is a possible option. However, much more research is required to refine these modalities prior to expanding the offerings to very young patients as proven therapies[19].

Patient-centered Approach for Elective and Medical Oocyte Cryopreservation

Elective Egg Freezing

Around the globe, the demand for elective egg freezing (EEF) is growing. For example, in the United States between 2013 and 2018, the total number of egg freezing cycles for all forms of FP jumped from 5000 to 12 000, according to the most recent Society for Assisted Reproductive Technology statistics[6,8,20,21].

Oocyte cryopreservation, thanks to the successful introduction of the vitrification technique, has also gained increasing acceptance for healthy women who are hoping to preserve their reproductive potential[20,22,23]. Oocyte cryopreservation in healthy women has been called "social egg freezing," "nonmedical egg freezing," "elective oocyte cryopreservation," "elective FP," and "oocyte banking for anticipated gamete exhaustion." Given the ongoing lack of agreement on the best nomenclature, we suggested "EEF" be added to the glossary of accepted terms[6] because it may most closely mirror women's preferred usage. In a large-scale interview-based study among 150 women who had completed EEF through four American IVF clinics and three in Israel, the chapter authors and colleagues reported that the majority (85%) of women in the study were unpartnered, while 15% had partners at the time of EEF[6]. Six pathways to EEF were found among women without partners (being single, divorced, broken up, deployed overseas, single mother, or career planner), with career planning being the least common reason for EEF. Among women with partners, four pathways to EEF were found (relationship too new or uncertain, partner not ready to have children, partner refusing to have children, or partner having multiple partners). Therefore, partnership problems, not career planning, lead most women on pathways to EEF. These pathways should be recognized in fertility clinics when offering consultations and advice to women planning EEF[6,20].

Several other anonymous surveys have also provided evidence regarding age and reasons for women's EEF motivations. A survey of 183 women who had completed at least one cycle of EEF during the years 2005–2011 showed that 84% were age 35 or older, and 88% had completed at least one cycle of EEF because they lacked a partner[24]. Another survey of 86 women in Belgium found that women were 36.7 years of age on average, and the overwhelming majority, 81%, lacked partners[25]. Similarly, in Australia, a survey of 96 women described as "socioeconomically advantaged" – highly educated (89%), professionals (88%), who owned private health insurance (93%) – had completed EEF between 1999 and 2014. Of these, 48% were 38 years or older, 90% were unpartnered, and 94% had not returned to use their eggs because they were not interested in being single mothers[26].

Our recently published qualitative assessments of 150 women's (114 in the United States and 36 in Israel) specific life circumstances and pathways to EEF confirmed that highly educated professional women are postponing motherhood and resorting to EEF for lack of a suitable partner rather than for career planning [6,8]. The average age for EEF was 36, with about three-quarters of women in both countries pursuing EEF in their late thirties. Almost all women who froze their eggs in both countries were highly educated and were ethnically and racially diverse. Most women (85%) were without partners at the time of EEF. However, being "partnered" or "unpartnered" are not monolithic categories, especially in terms of motivation to pursue EEF. Women in both categories faced a variety of different life circumstances that led them on the path to EEF[8]. Most women lamented the shortage of eligible men, especially men of equal educational and professional backgrounds. In some cases, women had tried "dating down" to widen their partnership possibilities, but they reported that less educated or less successful men had often acted as though they were "intimidated." Without a partner, these highly educated professional women had turned to EEF, usually in their late thirties, to "buy time," while continuing to search for a partner with the hope of future marriage and motherhood.

Among the women without partners, 17% had been previously married and 12% were never married but had recently "broken up" from long-term relationships. Ex-husbands were variously described by women as being unfaithful, over-controlling, narcissistic, alcoholic, or asexual. In the breakups group the reasons were their partners did not want children or changed their minds about having children, or already had children and did not want more, or were significantly younger and not ready to have children[20].

Only six women had undertaken EEF on the eventual path to single motherhood. Five of these women froze their eggs first, then decided to become "single mothers by choice."

Most considered single motherhood a very difficult choice: a "last resort" or "plan B." Women often cited the high financial costs of raising a child alone, especially in expensive cities such as New York, San Francisco, or Tel Aviv. For others, single motherhood suggested "desperation" or "failure," and they rejected it out of hand. Whether this EEF-assisted pathway to single motherhood will continue to grow is uncertain, but in this study, it comprised a small category among unpartnered women with the financial means to raise a child on their own.

Only one woman described her path to EEF as a career strategy. At age 30, she was significantly younger than most women in the study and was clear in her interview that her decision to freeze her eggs had allowed her to focus on her new career.

Fifteen percent of the women in the study were partnered at the time of EEF. About half of these partnered women were in secure, stable relationships with men who wanted to have children. But, in most cases, male partners were not yet "ready" to become fathers, usually because they were completing their education, making significant career moves, or were significantly younger (e.g., 5–18 years) than their female partners. Among partnered women, deployment overseas (8%), either in the military or for humanitarian organizations, was another reason for resorting to EEF. These long-term deployments sometimes last up to three years. These women's postings were also often in difficult and dangerous locations, including war zones and refugee camps.

Even though this "men as partners" problem has been well defined in public health scholarship, rarely has it been articulated in the assisted reproduction literature, so it is important to recognize the magnitude and heterogeneity of partnership problems in these women's lives. In both the United States and Israel, highly educated, professional women were experiencing their reproductive lives as being in jeopardy. EEF was their "technological concession": a way of putting their reproduction "on hold" in the absence of stable relationships with men committed to marriage and family making. For women themselves, this "men as partners" problem and the resultant "need" for EEF may be experienced as difficult, frustrating, and emotionally wrenching.

Patient-centered Approach for FP

To date, no attention has been paid to the specific needs of patients choosing to undergo FP. This issue is particularly relevant for women choosing EEF, or how they, as single women under reproductive time pressure, use non-medical FP or under concerns for their cancer diagnosis (medical FP) experience their care and treatment[7,8,21]. Single EEF patients may feel a sense of isolation and loneliness in the couples-oriented world of IVF. Furthermore, women undertaking EEF may have specific needs and desires for patient-centered care as they navigate the various challenges of ovarian testing, stimulation, and retrieval on their own. The need for patient-centered clinical care has been well documented over the past decade and is now considered one of six key dimensions of quality care; the others being safety, effectiveness, timeliness, efficiency, and equity of access. The results of our recent study[8] following the conceptual framework of "patient-centered infertility care" identified two broad categories and 11 specific dimensions of patient-centered EEF care, which are (1) *system factors*: information, competence of clinic and staff, coordination and integration, accessibility, physical comfort, continuity and transition, and cost, and (2) *human factors*: attitude and relationship with staff, communication, patient involvement and privacy, and emotional support. Cost was a unique factor of importance in both countries, despite their different healthcare delivery systems[8]. Given this scenario, IVF clinicians who are counseling and performing EEF should be aware of, and sensitive to, women's many partnership issues that are leading them on diverse pathways to EEF. Furthermore, it is important to realize that EEF patients are usually alone when they enter the couples-oriented world of IVF. Thus, IVF clinics must prioritize patient-centered care for the growing numbers of single women seeking EEF around the world. Last, a brief ethical concept. It is important to protect, particularly EEF patients, from nonunified standards and promises of success fueled by entrepreneurs seeking to capitalize on women's fears of losing their reproductive chances if they do not "freeze their eggs" with statements such as "smart women freeze" during martini infomercial cocktail parties. It is ethically irresponsible not to provide full information and to encourage women to put inordinate faith in techniques that, while exciting and even liberating, have no guaranteed success rates and have very high costs often not covered by insurance. Doctors and clinics offering egg-freezing services should tell patients up front what they need to know. This includes the number of cycles it might take to yield enough eggs, the cost for each cycle of cryopreservation including the medications, the cost to store the eggs per year, the known and unknown success rates for egg freezing at various ages, the costs associated with the future use of the frozen eggs with ICSI, the potential risks like OHSS during the ovarian stimulation, and the chances that, at the end, the procedure may not work and there will be no baby. They should also be clear about the disposition of gametes in case of death, severe disability, occurrence or reoccurrence of a life-shortening fatal illness, and if a decision is made by the donor not to personally use frozen oocytes. Without an absolute trust, demand for transparency of results and for standardization of care, patients seeking EEF will continue to find themselves confused and, in many cases, disappointed[27].

Conclusion and Future Directions

Advances in gamete and tissue cryopreservation have made FP a real possibility for patients whose gonadal function is threatened by treatments such as chemotherapy and radiotherapy or by medical conditions that pose a high risk for POI. Undoubtedly, success with oocyte vitrification has opened the possibility for healthy single women to postpone their reproductive plans. There are, however, still some issues that need additional research for widening the FP options.

Of immediate concern is the *risk of reimplanting malignant cells* contained in cryopreserved ovarian cortex since current methods to screen malignant contamination have significant limitations. There is no method or molecular marker that has 100% sensitivity and specificity for cancer cells. Histology, immunohistochemistry, polymerase chain reaction (PCR), and xenografting to severe combined immunodeficient mice had been used to evaluate the presence of metastases in ovarian cortex and in acute leukemia patients, more than 50% of tissue examined showed malignant cells detected by PCR, cautioning that reimplantation in these patients would be unsafe[28]. However, no malignant disease was found in the ovaries from leukemia patients in complete remission[29], suggesting that perhaps prior to offering OTC to patients with leukemia, they should undergo chemotherapy first.

Combination of ovarian tissue harvesting and immature oocyte collection: Cryopreservation of ovarian tissue may be combined with aspiration of small antral follicles, making it possible to freeze both ovarian tissue and isolated immature oocytes. Immature oocytes can be matured in vitro and then cryopreserved or used for IVF. The first live birth from a cryopreserved embryo obtained from an in vitro matured oocyte collected after oophorectomy was reported in 2014[30]. A retrospective cohort study of 255 cancer patients undergoing FP demonstrated significantly more oocytes, more MII oocytes, and better maturation rate by performing oocyte retrieval before ovarian resection for cryopreservation[31]. Although the potential benefits regarding pregnancy results and long-term follow-up data are still lacking, the combined approach allows more flexibility and more FP options to the patients.

Isolation of primordial follicles and in vitro maturation: Primordial follicles represent >90% of the total follicular reserve and show high cryotolerance. Small size of primordial follicles greatly facilitates penetration of cryoprotectant, and the oocyte it contains has a relatively inactive metabolism, as well as a lack of meiotic spindle, zona pellucida, and cortical granules[32]. For a patient who has a high risk of ovarian metastases, isolation of primordial follicles followed by in vitro folliculogenesis and subsequent cryopreservation of either mature oocytes or embryos could be an alternative to tissue reimplantation for FP.

The ability to develop human oocytes from the earliest follicular stages through to maturation and fertilization in vitro would revolutionize FP practice. This has been achieved in mice where in vitro grown (IVG) oocytes from primordial follicles have resulted in the production of live offspring. However, developing IVG systems to support complete development of human oocytes has been more difficult because of still poorly understood cellular checkpoints during in vivo oogenesis and differences in maturation timing and follicle size. Very recently, a dynamic three-step culture system that supports the activation and growth of human primordial follicles and oocyte growth outwith the large follicular environment up to metaphase II oocytes has been developed[33].

Another approach under investigation is transplanting a suspension of isolated primordial follicles. The transplantation of frozen-thawed isolated primordial follicles has been successfully achieved in mice, yielding normal offspring[34]. For human primordial follicles, however, mechanical isolation is not possible due to their size and the fibrous and dense ovarian stroma. Enzymatic digestion with Collagenase or Liberase has been used to isolate highly viable follicles with an unaltered morphology and ultrastructure[35]. Using the xenografting model, it has been shown that isolated human primordial follicles were able to survive and grow in vivo one week after xenografting in nude mice[36]. This study also showed massive in vivo follicular activation after the transplantation of isolated follicles. Further investigations revealed the potential for long-term survival of isolated human primordial follicles after xenografting, and subsequent development into antral follicles after FSH administration. Although this approach appeared promising, integrity assessment of human oocytes retrieved from cryopreserved ovarian tissue after xenotransplantation demonstrated that many oocytes grown in host animals and further matured in vitro had aberrant microtubule organization and chromatin patterns. Due to safety and ethical concerns, currently xenotransplantation to mature human ovarian follicles is not allowed in clinical practice.

Finally, we began experimenting in vitro whole ovine ovary perfusion to induce in vitro folliculogenesis. After 36 and 48 hours of perfusion (hMG and hCG) follicular growth and oocyte retrieval was demonstrated. In addition, this work could also be employed in "treating in vitro" with chemotherapy ovarian tissue from leukemia patients and purging it from potential seeds of cancer cells prior to cryopreservation[37].

References

1. Horner MJ, Ries LAG, Krapcho M et al. National Cancer Institute. SEER Cancer Statistics Review 1975–2006. https://seer.cancer.gov/archive/csr/1975_2006/index.html#contents

2. Kim SS, Donnez J, Barri P, Pellicer A, Patrizio P, Rosenwaks Z, et al. ISFP Recommendations for Fertility Preservation in Patients with Lymphoma, Leukemia, and Breast Cancer. *J Assist Reprod Genet.* 2012; 29(**6**): 465–8.

3. Lee SJ, Schover LR, Partridge AH, Patrizio P, Wallace WH, Hagerty K, et al. American Society of Clinical Oncology Recommendations on Fertility Preservation in Cancer Patients. *J Clin Oncol.* 2006; 24(**18**): 2917–31.

4. International Society Fertility Preservation Working Group. Update on fertility preservation from the Barcelona International Society for Fertility Preservation-ESHRE-ASRM 2015 expert meeting: Indications, results and future perspectives. *Fertil Steril.* 2017; 108(**3**): 407–15.

5. Cobo A, García-Velasco JA. Why All Women Should Freeze Their Eggs. *Clin Obstetr Gynecol.* 2016; 28: 206–10.

6. Inhorn MC, Birenbaum-Carmeli D, Birger J, Westphal LM, Doyle J, Gleicher N, et al. The Socio-Demographic of Elective Egg Freezing: A Binational Analysis of Fertility Preservation Among Unpartnered Healthy Women. *RBE.* 2018; 16(**1**): 70–81.

7. Inhorn MC, Birenbaum-Carmeli D, Westphal, LM, Doyle J, Gleicher N, Meirow D, et al. Medical Egg Freezing: The Importance of a Patient-Centered Approach to Fertility Preservation. *JARG.* 2018; 35(**1**): 49–59.

8. Inhorn MC, Birenbaum-Carmeli D, Westphal LM, Doyle J, Gleicher N, Meirow D, et al. Patient-Centered Elective Egg Freezing: A Binational Qualitative Analysis of Women's Quality-of-Care Desires. *JARG.* 2019.

9. Oktay K, Harvey BE, Partridge AH, Quinn GP, Reinecke J, Taylor HS, et al. Fertility Preservation in Patients with Cancer: ASCO Clinical Practice Guideline Update. *J Clin Oncol.* 2018; 36(**19**): 1994–2001.

10. Wallace WH, Thomson AB, Saran F, Kelsey TW. Predicting Age of Ovarian Failure After Radiation to a Field That Includes the Ovaries. *Int J Rad Oncol Biol Phys.* 2005; 62(**3**): 738–44.

11. Farber LA, Ames JW, Rush S, Gal D. Laparoscopic Ovarian Transposition to Preserve Ovarian Function Before Pelvic Radiation and Chemotherapy in a Young Patient with Rectal Cancer. *Med Gen Med.* 2005; 7: 66–71.

12. ASRM. Fertility Preservation and Reproduction in Patients Facing Gonadotoxic Therapies: An Ethics Committee Opinion. *Fertil Steril.* 2018; 110; 380–6.

13. Cobo A, García-Velasco JA, Domingo J, Remohí J, Pellicer A. Is Vitrification of Oocytes Useful for Fertility Preservation for Age-Related Fertility Decline and in Cancer Patients? *Fertil Steril.* 2013; 99(**6**): 1485–95.

14. Goldman KN, Noyes NL, Knopman JM, McCaffrey C, Grifo JA. Oocyte Efficiency: Does Live Birth Differ When Analyzing Cryopreserved and Fresh Oocytes on a Per Oocyte Basis? *Fertil Steril.* 2013; 100(**3**): 712–17.

15. Rienzi L, Cobo A, Paffoni A, Scarduelli C, Capalbo A, Vajta G, et al. Consistent and Predictable Delivery Rates After Oocyte Vitrification: An Observational Longitudinal Cohort Multicentric Study. *Hum Reprod.* 2012; 27(**6**): 1606–12.

16. Jensen AK, Macklon KT, Fedder J, Ernst E, Humaidan P, Andersen CY. 86 Successful Births and 9 Ongoing Pregnancies

Worldwide in Women Transplanted with Frozen-Thawed Ovarian Tissue: Focus on Birth and Perinatal Outcome in 40 of These Children. *J Assist Reprod Genet.* 2017; 34: 325–36.

17. Donnez J, et al. Restoration of Ovarian Function After Orthotopic (Intraovarian and Periovarian) Transplantation of Cryopreserved Ovarian Tissue in a Woman Treated by Bone Marrow Transplantation for Sickle Cell Anaemia: Case Report. *Hum Reprod.* 2006; 21(**1**): 183–8.

18. Borgstrom B, et al. Fertility Preservation in Girls with Turner Syndrome: Prognostic Signs of the Presence of Ovarian Follicles. *J Clin Endocrinol Metab.* 2009; 94(**1**): 74–80.

19. Patrizio P, Butt S, Caplan A. Ovarian Tissue Preservation and Future Fertility: Emerging Technologies and Ethical Considerations. *J Natl Cancer Inst Monogr.* 2005; 34: 107–10.

20. Inhorn MC, Birenbaum-Carmeli D, Westphal LM, Doyle J, Gleicher N, Meirow D, et al. Ten Pathways to Elective Egg Freezing. *JARG.* 2018; 35(**8**): 1277–83.

21. Inhorn MC, Birenbaum-Carmeli D, Patrizio P. Medical Egg Freezing and Cancer Patients' Hope: Fertility Preservation at the Intersection of Life and Death. *Soc Sci Med.* 2017; 195: 25–33.

22. Schon SB, Shapiro M, Gracia C, Senapati S. Medical and Elective Fertility Preservation: Impact of Removal of the Experimental Label from Oocyte Cryopreservation. *J Assist Reprod Genet.* 2017; 34: 1207–15.

23. Potdar N, Gelbaya TA, Nardo A. Oocyte Vitrification in the 21st Century and Post-Warming Fertility Outcomes: A Systematic Review and Meta-Analysis. *Reprod BioMed Online.* 2014; 29: 159–76.

24. Hodes-Wertz B, Druckenmiller S, Smith M, Noyes N. What Do Reproductive-Age Women Who Undergo Oocyte Cryopreservation Think About the Process As a Means to Preserve Fertility? *Fertil Steril.* 2014; 100: 1343–9.

25. Stoop D, Maes E, Polyzos NP, Verheyen G, Tournaye H, Nekkebroeck J. Does Oocyte Banking for Anticipated Gamete Exhaustion Influence Future Relational and Reproductive Choices? A Follow-Up of Bankers and Non-Bankers. *Hum Reprod.* 2015; 30: 338–44.

26. Hammarberg K, Kirkman M, Pritchard N, Hickey M, Peate M, McBain J, et al. Reproductive Experiences of Women Who Cryopreserved Oocytes for Non-Medical Reasons. *Hum Reprod.* 2017; 32: 575–81.

27. Patrizio P, Molinari E, Caplan AL. Ethics of Medical and Non-Medical Oocyte Cryopreservation. *Curr Opin Endocrinol Diabetes Obes.* 2016; 23(**6**): 470–5.

28. Dolmans MM, et al. Reimplantation of Cryopreserved Ovarian Tissue from Patients with Acute Lymphoblastic Leukemia Is Potentially Unsafe. *Blood.* 2010; 116(**16**): 2908–14.

29. Greve T, et al. Cryopreserved Ovarian Cortex from Patients with Leukemia in Complete Remission Contains No Apparent Viable Malignant Cells. *Blood.* 2012; 120(**22**): 4311–16.

30. Prasath EB, et al. First Pregnancy and Live Birth Resulting from Cryopreserved Embryos Obtained from in Vitro Matured Oocytes After Oophorectomy in an Ovarian Cancer Patient. *Hum Reprod.* 2014; 29(**2**): 276–8.

31. Hourwitz A, et al. Combination of Ovarian Tissue Harvesting and Immature Oocyte Collection for Fertility Preservation Increases Preservation Yield. *Reprod Biomed Online.* 2015; 31(**4**): 497–505.

32. Smitz JE, Cortvrindt RG. The Earliest Stages of Folliculogenesis in Vitro. *Reproduction.* 2002; 123(**2**): 185–202.

33. McLaughlin M, Albertini DF, Wallace WHB, Anderson RA, and Telfer EE. Metaphase II Oocytes from Human Unilaminar Follicles Grown in a Multistep

Culture System. *Mol Hum Reprod*. 2018; 24(**3**): 135–42.

34. Donnez J, Dolmans MM. Fertility Preservation in Women. *New Engl J Med*. 2017; 377: 1657–65.

35. Dolmans MM, et al. Evaluation of Liberase, a Purified Enzyme Blend, for the Isolation of Human Primordial and Primary Ovarian Follicles. *Hum Reprod*. 2006; 21(**2**): 413–20.

36. Dolmans MM, et al. Development of Antral Follicles After Xenografting of Isolated Small Human Preantral Follicles. *Reprod Biomed Online*. 2008; 16(**5**): 705–11.

37. Patrizio P, Milenkovich M, Loi P, Levi Setti PE, Arav A. New Strategies in Fertility Preservation: Freeze/Dry (Lyophilization) of Oocytes, Stem Cells and Chromosomes and in Vitro Whole Organ Perfusion. *JARG*. 2014; 31(**1**): 7–20.

Patient Retention, Nursing Retention: The Importance of Empathic Communication and Nursing Support

Alice D Domar

Introduction

The relationship between emotional health and infertility is a complex one. A hundred years ago, it was assumed that most, if not all, cases of infertility were due to issues with the female partner, and that psychiatric conditions were a significant contributor or even the cause of infertility. With the advent of more sophisticated diagnostic technology, the pendulum swung almost entirely in the opposite direction. The cause of infertility was attributed solely to organic causes in one or both partners, and any impact of emotional health was dismissed. Researchers even concluded as recently as the early 2000s that infertile women were no more distressed than fertile women, denied any impact of stress on fertility, and disregarded the possibility that psychological interventions could increase fertility. In addition, until 15 years ago, patient treatment termination was attributed to two causes: financial limitations and physician recommendation due to poor prognosis, also called active censoring. However, a series of studies published in 2004[1] determined that active censoring was uncommon and, in fact, the primary reason why insured patients dropped out of treatment was stress.

Nurses who work with infertility patients have to take on a number of roles, including financial counselor, therapist, and crisis counselor, as well as communicating complex treatment protocols. Much of their time is spent not with face-to-face patient contact, as they were trained, but instead over the telephone. Although many infertility clinics have nurses who have been on staff for decades, that trend is decreasing. The turnover rate for nurses in the REI field appears to be increasing rapidly, leading to patient dissatisfaction, rising stress levels of other nurses, and increased clinic costs for the recruitment and training of new nurses.

This chapter will address the issue of retention with both patients and nurses, which are likely intertwined since, as the stress levels of patients rise, theoretically so would their nurses'. And hypothetically, although there is no research to date to prove it, intervening to decrease the stress levels of patients could well not only increase patient retention but also have a positive impact on the stress levels of their nurses, which may lead to a decrease in turnover.

Patient Retention

Stress and Infertility

Prior to tackling the issue of patient retention, one needs to understand *why* patients drop out of treatment and *which* patients are the most likely to make that decision. For uninsured patients, finances are the primary reason why patients cannot initiate or continue with infertility treatment. However, for patients with financial resources and/ or insurance coverage, the emotional burden of that treatment is the most commonly cited reason for dropping out[2]. *Treatment termination* is defined as the decision to stop receiving infertility treatment despite a favorable prognosis where payment is not an issue.

In Israel, couples are covered by national health insurance to continue ART until they have two children, yet not all couples continue care. In a recent study of women under the age of 35, where 34% discontinued treatment[2], psychological burden was the most commonly cited reason for discontinuation, followed by lost hope of success; both of which reflect the distress caused by treatment. In a larger study in the United States[3], in a state which has a six-cycle mandated insurance coverage plan, of the women who terminated treatment, 40% reported that more treatment would have been too stressful. When these participants were asked more about their stress level, the top sources of stress were the feeling that they had already given IVF their best chance of success, feeling too stressed to continue, and infertility was taking too high a toll on their relationship.

Stress is in fact a significant factor for infertility patients. It is well known that women who are depressed are the least likely to initiate treatment. And, despite the impression of 15 years ago that infertility had a benign impact on psychological status, patients in treatment actually report high levels of distress. In a large recent study of both men and women who were receiving care in clinics in California, 56% of women and 32% of men scored in the clinical range for symptoms of depression and 76% of women and 61% of men scored in the clinical range for anxiety[4].

Despite the knowledge that distress is the most commonly cited reason for treatment termination and precludes treatment initiation, obviously not every distressed patient drops out of treatment. Thus, identifying which patients are the most likely to drop out would allow for pinpointing interventions at those most at risk. Research shows that risk factors for discontinuation include *female depression, poorer prognosis, longer duration of infertility, and higher parity*[5]. One cannot change prognosis, infertility duration, or parity. One can, however, treat stress.

Treating Stress

There have been dozens of RCTs on various psychological interventions designed to treat the distress reported by individuals and couples experiencing infertility. Unfortunately, these trials have included almost exclusively women already being seen at an infertility clinic. Thus, women who are not seeing an infertility specialist and men are vastly underrepresented.

In the largest most recent meta-analysis on the efficacy of psychological interventions with infertile women[6], 39 eligible studies were included on a total of 2746 women and men. The results were as follows: "statistically significant and robust overall effects" for both clinical pregnancy and combined negative psychological symptoms, which included depression, anxiety, stress, and marital function. There were no significant differences between cognitive behavioral therapy (CBT), mind body interventions (MBIs), and other forms of treatment, but the authors concluded that CBT and MBIs could be particularly efficacious. Other meta-analyses have included fewer trials, but most have come to the same conclusions in terms of the impact; structured interventions that provide specific skills acquisition to increase coping and reduce stress lead to decreases in psychological symptoms, specifically anxiety and depression. CBT has been highlighted more than other forms of intervention.

Preventing Treatment Termination

If one accepts the theory that stress is the leading contributor to insured patient dropout behavior, and that psychological interventions, specifically CBT, lead to decreases in distress, then it would be logical to assume that these interventions should also be associated with increases in patient retention.

Unfortunately, there is minimal research in this area. Only one study could be located through a literature review. In this study, 166 insured women were recruited prior to commencing their first IVF cycle[7]. Participants randomized to the intervention group received a packet in the mail, which contained a cognitive-coping and relaxation intervention (CCRI). The control participants received routine control (RC). The CCRI included two components: positive reappraisal coping and relaxation. The positive reappraisal intervention was a series of ten statements, all focused on infertility and its treatment, which encouraged the reader to think more about the positive aspects of their situation and to dwell less on recurrent negative thought patterns. There was one set for the stimulation phase of the ART cycle and one set for the waiting phase. In addition, the packet included instructions on relaxation; for the stimulation phase there were instructions on how to do "mini" relaxations and for the waiting phase, the packet included a guided CD on breath focus, meditation, and autogenic training.

All participants were followed for one year. In the CCRI group, 5.5% discontinued care compared to a 15.2% rate in the RC group. In addition, the CCRI participants engaged in significantly more positive reappraisal coping, an improved quality of life, less anxiety, and positively rated the intervention for ease of use, helpfulness, and the perception of stress reduction. There were no differences in pregnancy rates between the two groups.

Communicating with Patients

Physician/patient communication is a vital aspect of patient care. Many patient satisfaction surveys reveal that patients are highly sensitive to the communication style of their physician and this may impact a patient's decision on whether or not to initiate or continue with treatment. The ability of the physician to connect with patients is often revealed at the first visit, so connecting with patients at that visit is vital. In one study in Europe, 6% of patients did not return after that first visit[8]. In fact, half the patients dropped out before any treatment was initiated. Research has shown that unempathetic physicians are the most common complaint among infertility patients[9].

Infertility patients have a strong need to be understood and accepted by their physician, a concept called empathy. Empathic communication requires that the physician understand the patient's point of view and effectively communicate that they understand it, as well as tuning into the emotional state of the patient to establish trust. A physician can tell a patient that their pregnancy test was negative by simply saying, "your pregnancy test was negative," or a physician can be empathetic and say it in a different way: "I am so sorry to tell you that your pregnancy test was negative. I know this was not the outcome you were hoping for and that this may well feel incredibly disappointing. I am feeling so sad for you. When you are ready, I would love to sit down with you to talk about this cycle, and together see what we can plan for future, hopefully successful, treatment."

An infertility center in Spain recognized the need to improve their physicians' abilities in empathetic communication in an effort to keep patients from switching to other infertility clinics[9]. The focus was on the first patient visit: 1281 patients reported on their satisfaction with their physician after that first visit. Thirteen physicians then attended 14 hours of training over two days. The training included sessions on empathy, emotional intelligence, and verbal and nonverbal communication. Exercises included role-playing, active listening, and discovering one's own personal behavioral style. Two months after the training, 895 new patients reported on their satisfaction with their physician after the first visit. There were statistically significant positive increases on all aspects of physician assessment: information, dynamic, time, interaction, and professionalism. In addition, all the participating physicians were highly receptive to and satisfied with the training experience. Unfortunately, the study did not follow patients, so the impact of the training on patient compliance, emotional distress, and pregnancy rates is unknown.

Patient Retention: Summary and Suggestions for the Future

Individuals and couples who are experiencing infertility report high levels of stress. Many have clinical levels of anxiety and depression. Depression in women precludes them coming in to see an infertility specialist for a first visit and is a major contributor to their decision to not initiate or to terminate treatment. In addition, the psychological burden of treatment is the most common reason given why insured patients drop out of ART. Thus, distress leads to fewer individuals coming to an infertility clinic, proceeding to treatment, and staying in treatment until a viable pregnancy is established.

Research has firmly established that psychological interventions are associated with significant decreases in distress and most studies also show increases in pregnancy rates. Interventions with a CBT or mind/body focus appear to be the most efficacious. In addition, at least one RCT has shown that women who are provided with CBT and relaxation training experience less distress and are less likely to drop out of treatment.

It seems incredibly obvious that providing patients with stress-reducing skills is an obvious solution to the retention issue, yet it is rare for an infertility clinic to provide these opportunities. Yet papers published in 2012 and 2013 carefully outlined what could be easily implemented to reduce the treatment burden[10,11]. These suggestions included:

- screening patients for distress and referring at risk patients to an MHP prior to treatment
- creating educational materials to prepare patients adequately
- providing patients with easily accessible psychological counseling and coping interventions
- ensuring that the partner is included and involved
- simplifying treatment protocols
- integrating psychological support into patient daily care
- training physicians and staff on communication and interaction skills
- promoting shared decision-making
- changing/modifying areas that cause distress to patients
- supporting/educating patients on changing negative lifestyle habits
- creating ways to support patients who experience negative cycles
- accepting that, for some patients, treatment termination is their best choice

Research shows that supporting patients to complete their covered IVF cycles would result in far higher cumulative pregnancy rates as well as increases in cycles per year for clinics. Thus, creating initiatives to decrease patient stress would be a win–win. Patients would experience less distress, they would undergo more cycles, they would be more likely to conceive, and clinics would be busier.

Nursing Retention

Stress and the REI Nurse

Nurses play a vital role in the care of infertility patients. As previously mentioned, nurses wear a lot of different hats in many clinics. In addition to traditional nursing in the office, operating room and postanesthesia care unit (PACU) – and some nurses carry out all these roles – nurses also may do blood draws, vaginal ultrasounds, IUIs, and ETs, while simultaneously offering counseling, travel advice, financial information, and conflict resolution. In addition, even though their training involved in-person nursing care, in this field much of what nurses do is provide instructions and information to patients over the telephone. And this information tends to be complicated and tailored to each patient, and the patient population is highly anxious, does not retain information well, complains more, expects more, expresses dissatisfaction with their care, and frequently tends to ask the same questions over and over. In larger practices, one nurse may handle upwards of 100 telephone calls a day. Nurses spend far more time with patients than anyone else in the infertility clinic.

REI nursing is incredibly complex. It is estimated that, on average, it takes a year to train a new nurse before she or he is competent and comfortable. However, according to the 2017 survey of the Nursing Professional Group (NPG) of ASRM, only 18% of nurses participated in a formal training program. The vast majority of nurses reported learning through observation and only 45% received a formal orientation. The stress factor of nurses is described in the box.

Results from the 2016 NPG ASRM survey

- More than 80% of nurses responded that their workload had increased over the previous year
- More than 70% of nurses responded that their stress levels had increased over the previous year
- Most common reason why stress levels had increased: increased patient volume, increased workload
- More than 70% of nurses experienced symptoms of burnout
- More than 60% of nurses experienced compassion fatigue
- Most common suggestions to reduce burnout: better work/life balance, bonuses, more recognition

Compassion fatigue is the result of a caregiver trying their best to meet the overwhelming demands of stressed patients. It can lead not only to multiple physical and psychological symptoms in the caregiver but also to decreasing productivity and increasing turnover[12]. The most common symptoms of compassion fatigue are in Table 11.1. There has been a lot of research on factors that can impact compassion fatigue, nursing dissatisfaction, and turnover; none of it, however, on infertility nurses. In two recent systematic reviews, the most common factors included administrative support, salary, autonomy, meaningful work, adequate staffing, teamwork/cohesion, and job stress [13,14].

Because nurses spend so much time communicating with their infertility patients, they may well develop an emotional closeness. When patients are feeling anxious and upset, their nurses may begin to feel that way as well. However, drawing the nurse into the patient's emotional turmoil can negatively impact the nurse's well-being, so many nurses try to emotionally distance themselves from their patients, which the patients may become aware of. And resent. In one of the first studies on REI nurse well-being[15], 15

Table 11.1 Compassion fatigue symptoms

Work related	Psychological
Avoidance of working with specific patients	Irritability
Lack of job satisfaction	Anxiety/depression/lability
Decrease in capacity to express or feel empathy	Increase in mistakes
Increase in number of sick days taken	Resentment
Physical	
Sleep issues/fatigue	
Gastrointestinal symptoms	
Headaches/back pain/muscle aches	
Palpitations, shortness of breath	

nurses from New Zealand were interviewed about their experiences. As expected, nurses reported spending almost half their day speaking to patients on the telephone. Their roles included emotional support, information provision, interpreting medical data, and advocating for the patients with their physicians. Nurses needed to "hold together" to balance both the needs of their patients as well as their own well-being. The authors concluded that nurses need training and support, a place where personal issues can be safely addressed, debriefing opportunities, guidance on maintaining boundaries, and adequate professional development opportunities.

The issue of nurse training in providing emotional support versus the clinic's responsibility to provide patients with other resources to decrease their distress is receiving more recent interest[16]. The question is, do nurses have a responsibility to psychologically counsel their patients in addition to their other roles?

In one of the only studies to have queried health-care professionals who work in the REI field[17], respondents reported on the challenges of working with infertility patients. Unfortunately, the response rate for the study was only 8.9% and only 7% of the respondents were nurses. However, there were a number of themes that were identified which match the nursing reports in the literature. The most common stressors were inadequate amount of time to do one's job, clinic management issues, work environment/challenging administration, too high patient expectations, the demands of patient counseling, and patient misinformation. Suggested solutions included *training in patient communication as well as dealing with challenging patients and patient situations, handling teamwork issues, workload planning, handling complaints, and unexpected events.*

As previously mentioned, there is likely a strong relationship between patient and nurse stress levels. Anxious patients are likely to lead to anxious nurses. And vice versa. Thus, it is anticipated that satisfied nurses may lead to increases in patient satisfaction with care. In fact, in research with 2596 army nurses, nursing satisfaction was the most consistent predictor of increases in patient satisfaction, as well as decreases in reported adverse events[18].

Methods to Lower Stress in the REI Nurse

No studies that were dedicated to treating the stress levels of infertility nurses could be located in the literature. There was one study that investigated the impact of training nurses in a form of care called the "Theory of Human Caring"[19]. This theory is based on the idea that patients cannot be treated as objects: their care requires that caregivers be "present, attentive, conscious, and intentional." The study was an RCT with 105 Turkish infertility patients. Half were randomized to be cared for by nurses who focused on four areas: developing and sustaining a caring, trusting relationship, becoming aware of the distress level of the patient, reaching for solutions/problem solving, and teaching relaxation to enhance coping. It was an intensive intervention; the intervention patients received four 45–90-minute interviews with their nurse who applied a variety of techniques including active listening, empathy, reassurance, empowerment, and coaching in positive thinking. These patients also received training through a booklet on relaxation techniques and each interview ended with a relaxation accompanied by "relaxing music, candlelight, and lavender and rose scents." Each patient could also have a 5–10-minute back massage after her interview. The control participants received routine nursing care. Not surprisingly, the intervention patients reported significant decreases in distress, and increases in self-efficacy and adjustment. The practicality of this intervention, however, would preclude its widespread dissemination.

Strategies to Reduce Nursing Turnover

There is some research on stress reduction strategies for nurses in general, although many studies are of poor quality. In one literature review, the only two strategies that had some efficacy in reducing nursing turnover were preceptorship of newly graduated nurses and increased leadership for group cohesion[20]. In two recent studies, it was reported that a "purposeful interprofessional team training" led to higher job satisfaction ratings[21] and that including nurses in decision-making and improving their well-being led to decreases in turnover intentions[22].

Unfortunately, there is no available research on interventions to reduce infertility nurse turnover. However, the same approach to other forms of nursing could well be tried. In addition, *more formal training, which includes a thorough explanation of the patient perspective of the infertility experience, as well as peer mentoring, an increased sense of control, formal recognition programs, specific incentives based on performance, and regular opportunities for nurses to debrief and learn stress reduction strategies* are recommended.

Tackling the Challenge of Retention in Both Patients and Nurses: The Role of the MHP

High distress levels in infertility patients lead to a variety of negative consequences: anxiety and depressive symptoms are unpleasant for the patient to experience, distressed patients are challenging for the nurse to care for, the patients are more likely to drop out of treatment, and the nurses frequently reach a point where they decide to pursue employment elsewhere[23].

In a special report from ESHRE[24], it was recommended that patient counseling be provided by MHPs, rather than the medical team, for many reasons, including appropriate screening of distress levels (patients may "fake good" for their physician or nurse in an attempt to continue treatment), private opportunities to discuss sexual issues, expert counseling on marital problems, as well as an unbiased sounding board to contemplate stopping treatment. At the very least, all patients should be offered a visit with an MHP, especially after an unsuccessful cycle.

An MHP can provide a triple role of efficacy: treating and even preventing distress with patients, which theoretically leads to less distress in nurses, and simultaneously providing similar stress reduction services to nurses. An embedded MHP can provide crisis counseling for patients as well as nurses and, in addition, can offer regular opportunities for the nursing staff to learn how to better communicate with patients as well as how to better care for themselves in their work setting.

At Boston IVF, there are numerous programs designed to treat and prevent distress in both patients and nurses. There is a psychologist on site daily to be called in for crises in the clinic as well as the PACU and ultrasound rooms. All patients with an abnormal prenatal ultrasound are invited to speak to a psychologist within one hour of their scan. Every patient with an unsuccessful treatment cycle is offered a free 30-minute session with one of the psychologists, and there is a psychologist available for after-hour telephone consults for emergencies. These are all in addition to regularly scheduled individual and couples counseling appointments, a mind/body program, acupuncture 365 days/year, and nutritional counseling. For nurses, there is crisis counseling available daily as well as regularly scheduled "stress lunches" where challenging patient situations are presented and debriefed, and stress management training takes place, as well as training in empathetic communication.

Conclusion: Tackling Retention in the REI Clinic

The key to increasing patient and nurse retention involves numerous factors including money, control, and stress. Teaching patients and nurses strategies to decrease their stress levels may well offer a significant solution to the retention challenge. The question remains, however, how to best do this in a way that is cost-effective, palatable to both, and efficient. Strategies such as mobile apps, online instruction, and staff training need to be explored and implemented to reach the mutual goals of calmer patients, less harried nurses, higher patient volume, and more healthy babies.

References

1. Domar AD. Impact of Psychological Factors on Dropout Rates in Insured Infertility Patients. *Fertil Steril.* 2004; 81: 271–3.

2. Lande Y, Seidman DS, Maman E, Baum M, Hourvitz A. Why Do Couples Discontinue Unlimited Free IVF Treatments? *Gynecol Endocrinol.* 2015; 31: 233–6.

3. Domar AD, Rooney K, Hacker MR, Sakkas D, Dodge LE. Burden of Care Is the Primary Reason Why Insured Women Terminate in Vitro Fertilization Treatment. *Fertil Steril.* 2018; 109: 1121–6.

4. Pasch LA, Holley SR, Bleil ME, Shehab D, Katz PP, Adler NE. Addressing the Needs of Fertility Patients and Their Partners: Are They Informed of and Do They Receive Mental Health Services? *Fertil Steril.* 2016; 106: 209–15.

5. Pedro J, Sobral MP, Mesquita-Guimarães J, Leal C, Costa ME, Martins MV. Couples' Discontinuation of Fertility Treatments: A Longitudinal Study on Demographic, Biomedical, and Psychosocial Factors. *J Assist Reprod Genet.* 2017; 34: 217–24.

6. Frederiksen Y, Farver-Vestergaard I, Skovgard NG, Ingerslev HJ, Zachariae R. Efficacy of Psychosocial Interventions for Psychological and Pregnancy Outcomes in Infertile Woman and Men: A Systematic Review and Mate-Analysis. *BMJ Open.* 2015; 5: 1–18.

7. Domar AD, Gross J, Rooney K, Boivin J Exploratory Randomized Trial on the Effect of a Brief Psychological Intervention on Emotions, Quality of Life, Discontinuation, and Pregnancy Rates in in Vitro Fertilization Patients. *Fertil Steril.* 2015; 104: 440–51.

8. Brandes M, van der Steen JOM, Bokdam SB, Hamilton CJCM, de Bruin JP, Nelen WLDM, et al. When and Why Do Subfertile Couples Discontinue Their Fertility Care? A Longitudinal Cohort Study in a Secondary Care Subfertility Population. *Human Reprod.* 2009; 24: 3127–35.

9. Garcia D, Bautista O, Venereo L, Coll O, Vassena R, Vernaeve V. Training in Empathic Skills Improves the Patient-Physician Relationship During the First Consultation in a Fertility Clinic. *Fertil Steril.* 2013; 99: 1413–18.

10. Gameiro S, Boivin J, Domar AD. Optimal in Vitro Fertilization in 2020 Should Reduce Treatment Burden and Enhance Care Delivery for Patients and Staff. *Fertil Steril.* 2013; 100: 302–9.

11. Boivin J, Domar AD, Shapiro DB, Wischmann TH, Fauser BCJM, Verhaak C. Tackling Burden in ART: An

Integrated Approach for Medical Staff. *Hum Reprod*. 2012; 27: 941–50.

12. Lombardo B, Eyre C. Compassion Fatigue: A Nurse's Primer. *Online J Issues Nurs*. 2011; 16: 1–7.

13. Dilig-Ruiz A, MacDonald I, Demery VM, Vandyk A, Graham ID, Squires JE. Job Satisfaction Among Critical Care Nurses: A Systematic Review. *Int J Nurs Stud*. 2018; 88: 123–34.

14. Han RM, Carter P, Champion JD. Relationship Among Factors Affecting Advanced Practice Registered Nurses' Job Satisfaction and Intent to Leave: A Systematic Review. *J Am Assoc Nurse Pract*. 2018; 30: 101–13.

15. Payne D, Goedeke S. Holding Together: Caring for Clients Undergoing Assisted Reproductive Technologies. *J Adv Nurs*. 2007; 60: 645–53.

16. Wilson C, Leese B. Do Nurses and Midwives Have a Role in Promoting the Well-Being of Patients During Their Fertility Journey? A Review of the Literature. *Hum Fertil*. 2013; 16: 2–7.

17. Boivin J, Bunting L, Koert E, Chin ieng U, Verhaak C. Perceived Challenges of Working in a Fertility Clinic: A Qualitative Analysis of Work Stressors and Difficulties Working with Patients. *Hum Reprod*. 2017; 32: 403–8.

18. Perry SJ, Richter JP, Beauvais B. The Effects of Nursing Satisfaction and Turnover Cognitions on Patient Attitudes and Outcomes: A Three-Level Multisource Study. *Health Serv Res*. 2018; 53(**6**): 4943–69.

19. Arslan-Ozkan I, Okumus H, Buldukoglu K. A Randomized Controlled Trial of the Effects of Nursing Care Based on Watson's Theory of Human Caring on Distress, Self-Efficacy and Adjustment in Infertile Women. *J Adv Nurs*. 2013; 1801–12.

20. Halter M, Pelone F, Boiko O, Beighton C, Harris R, Gale J, et al. Interventions to Reduce Adult Nursing Turnover: A Systematic Review of Systematic Reviews. *Open Nurs J*. 2017; 11: 108–23.

21. Baik D, Zierler B. Job Satisfaction and Retention After an Interprofessional Team Intervention. *West J Nurs Res*. 2019; 41(**4**): 615–30.

22. Marques-Pinto A, Jesus EH, Mendes AMOC, Fronteira I, Roberto MS. Nurses' Intention to Leave the Organization: A Mediation Study on Professional Burnout and Engagement. *Span J Psychol*. 2018; 8(**21**): e32.

23. Domar AD. Creating a Collaborative Model of Mental Health Counseling for the Future. *Fertil Steril*. 2015; 104: 277–80.

24. Peterson B, Boivin J, Norre J, Smith C, Thorn P, Wischmann T. An Introduction to Infertility Counseling: A Guide for Mental and Medical Professionals. *J Assist Reprod Genet*. 2012; 29: 243–8.

Chapter 12

Patient-Centered IVF Care

Sofia Gameiro

The notion that health professionals should try to understand illness and its treatments from the patients' perspective instead of solely relying on scientific knowledge first emerged in the nursing profession during the 1960s[1]. It was only in the new millennium that this perspective came into use within infertility and assisted reproductive technology (ART), when the argument was made that patient centeredness was as important in defining high-quality ART as other treatment dimensions, such as effectiveness, efficiency, or safety[2]. Interest in understanding patients' views and experiences of treatment, as well as their expressed needs and preferences, has since been increasing steadily. Currently there is an understanding that health practitioners need to combine the best available evidence with patients' preferences and needs in all their clinical decision-making.

Patient-centered care (PCC) is care that respects and responds to individual patient preferences, needs, and values, and ensures that patient values guide all clinical decisions. In the last two decades, there has been great progress in working towards a more centered ART. First, research identified 11 PCC dimensions important to patients: information provision, competence of clinic and staff, coordination and integration, access to care, continuity and transition, and physical comfort are considered to be system factors (of the clinic), while respect, attitude of and relationship with staff, communication, patient involvement, and emotional support are considered to be human factors (of the staff) [3,4]. Data about which specific aspects within each dimension are more important, for which patient groups, during which stages of treatment, and at which clinical settings (e.g., geographical variation) are starting to appear but are still largely lacking. Second, infertility-specific measures to assess patients' experiences with care were developed, such as the patient-centeredness questionnaire (PCQ)-Infertility (see Table 12.2), which has been validated in different languages and can be modified to assess staff views on the care they provide. Third, probing into the relative value patients and staff attribute to PCC showed that staff underestimate the importance of PCC and that patients are willing to pay more and trade pregnancy rates to receive better PCC. Research also showed that patients and staff evaluated differently the quality of care provided at their clinics[5]. In the future, it will be important to better understand the underlying staff attitudes that explain this discrepancy, as well as the barriers that make it hard for clinics and staff to improve PCC. Fourth, research has also shown that some aspects of PCC are associated with patient well-being and quality of life[6,7], although so far there is only promising research supporting the claim that patients who receive better PCC are less likely to discontinue treatment[8,9]. Future steps must address the direction of causality in these relationships. Fifth, further conceptual development led to the distinction between PCC and patient-centered treatment (PCT). PCT refers to the valuing of the patient role in treatment-shared decision-making[10] and includes the dimensions of burden, time, effectiveness, potential risks, financial costs, and genetic parentage. Finally, a few complex interventions to increase PCC were evaluated but showed little promise so far[11]. Simultaneously, interventions focusing on single dimensions of PCC showed that improvements can be achieved[12]. It may be more feasible to try to create incremental change by focusing on one aspect of PCC at the time than to simultaneously address all aspects.

This chapter takes the view that it would also be useful to think about PCC in terms of what it aims to achieve. This view could provide clarity in terms of prioritizing change in care, understanding connections between the different PCC dimensions and why these are valued by patients, and designing future studies and interventions, including testing of specific hypotheses. We argue that PCC aims to achieve three important goals: (1) centeredness: respecting patients and their stated preferences, needs, and values, (2) engagement: empowering patients to share the management of infertility and its treatment with the fertility team, and (3) personalization: adapting care and treatment services to patients. Figure 12.1 illustrates these three goals and the PCC dimensions more closely related with each goal.

With a view to what should be considered optimal PCC in ART, this review puts forward a set of recommendations for researchers and health practitioners interested in working toward these three PCC goals. Table 12.1 presents a summary of the formulated recommendations. Table 12.2 lists available resources that may be useful for staff and clinics interested in following our recommendations.

Centeredness: Respecting Patients and Their Stated Preferences, Needs, and Values

Considerable research has been done to explore patients' needs and preferences regarding the way they are taken care of at clinics and their interactions with staff. Two reviews highlight the following aspects as being the most important to patients[3,13]:

- Being cared for by respectful, sensitive, and trustworthy staff members. This includes all staff members at fertility clinics, including office staff and, in particular, physicians.
- Positive attitude (e.g., being friendly) of, and interactions with, all staff members, and physicians in particular.

Table 12.1 Summary of recommendations per patient-centered care (PCC) goal

Goal of patient-centered care	Recommendations
Centeredness Respecting patients and their stated preferences, needs, and values	• Increase awareness of patients' preferences and train staff in centeredness
Engagement Empowering patients to share the management of infertility and its treatment with the fertility team	• Provide information • Promote empathetic care by offering staff access to personal narratives and views about infertility and ART • Promote patient self-care (stress, lifestyle, and compliance) • Promote and develop tools for shared decision-making
Personalization Adapting care and treatment services to patients (instead of patients to treatments and clinics)	• Involve patients in research and other initiatives to improve quality of care • Promote patient positive adjustment to unsuccessful fertility treatment

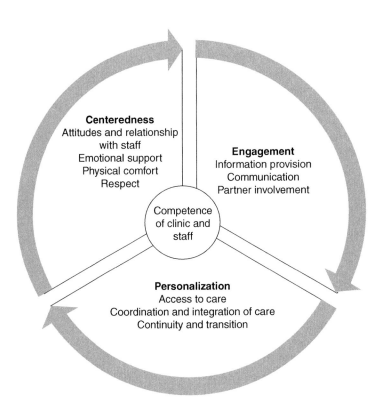

Figure 12.1 Three important aims (in bold) of patient-centered care (PCC) and their underlying dimensions. The arrows indicate the interdependence between the three PCC aims and their underlying dimensions. The dimension competence of clinic and staff is a requisite to all PCC provision.

- Responsiveness and sensitivity of staff toward the emotional impact of infertility and its treatment, as well as toward distinct needs related with patients' background and medical history.
- Provision of emotional support before, during, and after treatment, in particular by physicians and nurses and during the two-week waiting period for the pregnancy test.
- Opportunity for contact with prior patients, and access to patient support groups and to specialized psychosocial care (counseling, therapy).

Aspects related to the attitude of and relationship with staff are considered to be of higher priority than receiving emotional support[4].

Recommendations

Increase Awareness of Patients' Preferences and Train Staff in Centeredness

Centeredness is an important aspect for patients. Patients report that they are willing to sacrifice 10% of the pregnancy rate if that means being cared for by a friendly and interested physician (as compared with unfriendly, uninterested) and that lack of PCC is an important driver for them to stop treatment or continue it at a different clinic[14,15]. Staff attitudes seem to be particularly important for women, patients with lower education, and patients undergoing treatment for a longer time[14].

Poor interactions between ART professionals and patients are commonly reported in the literature[3,16] and the consequences include dissatisfaction with care and more medical malpractice suits. This may happen because staff are not fully aware of how important their attitude to patients is, lack knowledge about how to improve the quality of their interactions, or are highly time pressured by other job demands. It may also be that some patients' demands are too difficult to satisfy (e.g., immediate feedback to emails or calls). Whatever the reality is, research shows that staff are open to change and think that evaluating current practices, discussing these within the team, and receiving feedback and patient input would help them in this endeavor[14,17].

Multiple studies showed that interpersonal and communication skills can be learned and retained long term, and result in higher patient satisfaction[12] and benefits for staff themselves, such as higher perceived self-confidence and reduced burnout. A meta-analysis of 13 RCTs in other health conditions where the patient–staff relationship was manipulated showed that this results in a small but significant impact on patient subjective health outcomes (e.g., pain, quality of life, anxiety). These data show that there are evidence-based interventions available for clinics to invest in training their staff in centeredness as these should translate into better patient subjective well-being and satisfaction with care. These should be incorporated into all staff's continuous professional development. Research should also focus on conducting further efficacy testing of these interventions within the specific context of infertility and ART.

Staff's responsiveness and sensitivity is of particular importance when patients receive bad news, which is a common occurrence in infertility and ART, for instance,

Table 12.2 Resources available for staff and clinics

Increase awareness of patients' preferences and train staff in centeredness

SPIKES protocol to deliver bad news: Baile WF, Buckman R, Lenzi R, Glober G, Beale EA, Kudelka AP. SPIKES – A Six-Step Protocol for Delivering Bad News: Application to the Patient with Cancer. *Oncologist*. 2000; 5(**4**): 302–11.

Provide information

NHS. The Information Standard Principles.
www.england.nhs.uk/tis/about/

Promote empathetic care

Graphic novels:
– Knight P. *The Facts of Life*. Myriad. 2017.
– Potts P. *Good Eggs*. Harper. 2010.

DrawingOut method:
– https://www.drawingout.org

Patient co-produced booklets based on the DrawingOut method:

– Thorns and Flowers: Infertility Experiences of Black and Minority Ethnic Women.
https://drawingout.org/thorns-and-flowers-infertility-experiences-of-black-and-minority-ethnic-women/
– Experiences of endometriosis in Wales.
https://www.cardiff.ac.uk/__data/assets/pdf_file/0009/1319571/Boivin_Working_paper_Series_Endometriosis_in_Wales_16APR_2018.pdf
– Fertility Fest.
https://www.fertilityfest.com

Promote patient self-care

Patient questionnaires:
– COMPI Fertility Problem Stress Scales
  Sobral MP, Costa ME, Schimdt L, Martins MV. COMPI Fertility Problem Stress Scales is a Brief, Valid, and Reliable Tool for Assessing Stress in Patients Seeking Treatment. *Human Reproduction*. 2017; 32(**2**): 375–82.
– Fertility Problem Inventory
  Newton CR. The Fertility Problem Inventory: Measuring Perceived Infertility-related Stress. *Fertility and Sterility*. 1999; 72: 54–62.
– FertiQoL
  Boivin J, Takefman J, Braverman A. The Fertility Quality of Life (FertiQoL) Tool: Development and General Psychometric Properties. *Human Reproduction*. 2011; 26(**8**): 2084–91.
– PRCI
  Lancastle D, Boivin J. A Feasibility Study of a Brief Coping Intervention (PRCI) for the Waiting Period Before a Pregnancy Test During Fertility Treatment. *Human Reproduction*. 2008; 23: 2299–307.
– SCREENIVF
  Van Dongen AJ, Kremer JA, Van Sluisveld N, Verhaak CM, Nelen WL. Feasibility of Screening Patients for Emotional Risk Factors Before in Vitro Fertilization in Daily Clinical Practice: A Process Evaluation. *Human Reproduction*. 2012; 27(**12**): 3493–501.

Table 12.2 (cont.)

Promote and develop tools for shared decision-making

Option Grid decision aids.
https://health.ebsco.com/products/option-grid

Involve patients in research and other initiatives to improve quality of care

PCC questionnaires:
- PCQ-Infertility

  van Empel IWH, Aarts JWM, Cohlen BJ, Huppelschoten DA, Laven JSE, Nelen WL, Kremer JAM. Measuring Patient-Centeredness, the Neglected Outcome in Fertility Care: A Random Multicentre Validation Study. *Human Reproduction.* 2010; 25(**10**): 2516–26.
- Quality from the Patient Perspective (PPQ-IVF)

  Holter H, Sandin-Bojo, Gejervall A-L, Wikland M, Wilde-Larsson, Bergh C. Quality of Care in an IVF Programme from a Patient's Perspective: Development of a Validated Instrument. *Human Reproduction.* 2014; 29(**3**): 534–47.
- FertiQol – Treatment Module

  Boivin J, Takefman J, Braverman A. The Fertility Quality of Life (FertiQoL) Tool: Development and General Psychometric Properties. *Human Reproduction.* 2011; 26(**8**): 2084–91.

Guidance to involve patients in research:
- NHS. Involve. www.invo.org.uk/
- NIHR (2014). *Patient and public involvement in health and social care research: A handbook for researchers.* Online article. https://www.rds-yh.nihr.ac.uk/wp-content/uploads/2015/01/RDS_PPI-Handbook_2014-v8-FINAL-11.pdf
- AHRQ. Patient and Family Engagement. www.ahrq.gov/professionals/education/curriculum-tools/cusptoolkit/modules/patfamilyengagement/index.html
- AIR. Patient + Family Engagement in Healthcare. https://patientfamilyengagement.org

Promote patient-positive adjustment to unsuccessful fertility treatment

Fertility Network UK. More to Life.
http://fertilitynetworkuk.org/for-those-facing-the-challenges-of-childlessness/support/

receiving an infertility diagnosis or receiving news of stimulation, oocyte pickup, fertilization, and treatment failure. Thirty-seven percent and seventeen percent of patients experience unexpected emotional and physical reactions, respectively, when being informed about treatment outcome (e.g., not being able to sleep or stop crying). Those with a negative result are more likely to think that staff had better ways to communicate the news and help them react to the result. This is also one of the biggest perceived challenges of working in ART[17]. In sum, both staff and patients can benefit from staff improving their skills on this topic. One way to achieve this is by using a predefined protocol to share bad news. Indeed, it is known from other areas of health that, when physicians know how to proceed in these contexts, both staff and patients experience less stress. A recent study showed that ART professionals think a protocol to share bad news can be practical and useful[18]. Following a sensitive protocol may also help prevent extremely negative emotional reactions from patients, which are highly stressful and time consuming for staff. Another approach that some infertility staff welcome is to attend training workshops on how to share bad news[17]. Table 12.2 presents a well-known protocol to share bad news.

Engagement: Empowering Patients to Share The Management of Infertility and Its Treatment with The Fertility Team

The focus on engagement acknowledges that patients can play an important role in their own healthcare. This includes accessing and understanding health information, taking action that maximizes treatment success chances and decreases risk (self-care), and working together with clinicians to make treatment decisions (shared decision-making).

The PCC literature shows that patients value[3,13,19]:

- receiving written comprehensive and customized (i.e., personally relevant) information about different aspects of their treatment, including: diagnosis, treatment plan, treatment options and results, emotional implications of treatment, available support, and self-care options
- being given time to discuss the above listed issues with fertility staff
- fertility staff paying attention to their input
- both partners being explicitly involved in the treatment process (when applicable)
- being given the opportunity for shared decision-making

Recommendations

Provide information

There are many reasons why providing adequate preparatory information is essential. Besides being an ethical requirement for informed consent and the most valued PCC dimension, it increases compliance, reduces anticipatory anxiety and stress, increases patients' knowledge about treatment, and addresses their concerns[13]. Compared with other components of care such as complex interventions or counseling, it can be easier and more cost-effective to incorporate information provision in routine care via multiple media (clinics' websites, pamphlets, in person, and so on). Many scientific societies and regulatory bodies have stressed the importance of, and developed guidelines on, information provision (e.g., which, how)[13,20].

Notwithstanding, the reality is that information provision guidelines are not adhered to. For instance, in the United States, only 56% and 40% of private and academic clinics publish their success rates and only one in five explains how these are calculated. Very recently, the same was found for Australian and New Zealand clinics. Multiple studies have also shown that many information needs of patients are not met; for instance, how to access psychological resources, alternatives to IVF treatment, advantages and disadvantages of stopping treatment, or access to other parenting options. Fertility staff may be unable to provide information because of multiple job demands and lack of time[16]. Nonetheless, clinics cannot rely on patients finding information elsewhere. Indeed, studies show that patients use the Internet, but the quality of information available there varies greatly. Even when patients use expert forums, only 55% are satisfied with the clarifications they receive.

What is it that clinics can do to improve the quality of the information they provide? First, they can make sure that their websites comply with current guidelines and codes of practice; in particular in what concerns information about success rates. Second, they can develop quick guides explaining the diagnosis and treatment procedures offered and what they entail for patients (e.g., producing a sperm sample, single-ET). Third, they can develop information addressing the specific needs patients experience before, during, and after treatment (e.g., time away from work, two-week waiting period, reactions to a failed fertility treatment), which are now well documented[13]. Fourth, they can focus on the needs experienced by subgroups of patients (e.g., immigrants, ethnic, and sexual minorities, and so on). Fifth, clinics should be acquainted with standards developed to ensure the good quality of the information produced (see an example in Table 12.2). Such standards usually focus on issues such as using up-to-date, trustworthy evidence, ensuring patient understanding (e.g., accounting for language and health literacy), co-production of materials by patients and staff, friendly design, accessibility, regular reviews, and so on. Finally, clinics may want to consider when and how they deliver information. It may be time efficient to deliver information ahead of consultations, as staff can then better use consultation time to address patients' uncertainties and concerns. How to deliver information is also important, as studies show that patients do not always read posters or notice leaflets.

Promote Empathetic Care by Offering Staff Access to Personal Narratives and Views About Infertility and ART

If staff want to successfully involve patients in treatment, they need to have an in-depth understanding of how all patients experience treatment and of the needs and values that guide their treatment decisions. These are likely to vary across patient populations, depending on factors such as the clinical setting, ethnicity, citizenship status, sexuality, and so on. For instance, minority ethnic groups and immigrants have increased needs for information and experience barriers when communicating with staff (e.g., due to language and socio-cultural differences). Some minority ethnic groups may also be less receptive to some diagnostic and treatment procedures due to cultural or religious reasons. LGBTQ patients are often confronted with information framed for heterosexual couples only, which may not include procedures specific to their situation. Without awareness of specific needs and preferences staff cannot tailor care to meet these nor properly empower patients to manage their infertility and associated treatment.

Healthcare staff are more often trained on the scientific knowledge needed to treat infertility than on the kinds of empathetic knowledge relevant to the sensitive care of infertile patients. Multiple initiatives have been developed using innovative mediums to provide healthcare professionals with new insights into the personal experiences of diseases. Examples are presented in Table 12.2 and include graphic novels, patient co-produced comic booklets using the DrawingOut method[21], theater-based workshops[22], or art festivals. Instead of providing information, such initiatives tend to communicate the less visible aspects of patients' experiences in a simple but striking way that promotes visceral understanding alongside offering an esthetical and entertaining experience. Clinics can foster a policy of empathetic care by making these materials or initiatives accessible to their staff. Such materials can also be useful for patients wanting to learn more about their illness and connect with other affected people.

Promote Patient Self-Care

Clinics should support patients in increasing their self-care ability. In ART, self-care includes managing stress, adopting a healthy lifestyle, and capitalizing on cumulative pregnancy rates by undergoing treatment until pregnancy is achieved (unless recommended to stop). Patients experience stress during treatment because of the uncertainty of its outcome and particularly during the two-week waiting period. Self-care during this period can be promoted with the PRCI (see Table 12.2), a self-help tool that prompts positive reappraisal coping, helping patients to sustain coping until they get their treatment result. Patients can also benefit from knowing that, contrary to general belief, stress does not have a direct negative impact on the outcome of treatment[23,24]. Finally, fertility-specific distress and quality-of-life tools (e.g., SCREENIVF, FertiQoL, COMPI Fertility Problem Stress Scales, Fertility Problem Inventory: see Table 12.2) can be useful for patients to develop insight about their psychosocial vulnerabilities to treatment and discuss these, as well as suitable support strategies, with formal and informal carers in advance of treatment.

There is strong evidence showing the negative impact of female BMI and smoking on multiple fertility indicators such as time to conception, oligozoospermia or azoospermia, IVF success, and miscarriages. Staff need to be aware that a considerable number of patients have lifestyles that may affect their general and reproductive health and that they can assess this with self-administered tools[13]. This exercise could be the starting point for a conversation with patients about how their lifestyle choices may affect their parenthood aspirations. Patients at risk for a poor outcome can be encouraged to undergo lifestyle interventions. Diet- plus exercise-based interventions have proved successful in achieving weight loss and treatment-independent rates of pregnancy, but not live birth. It has recently been argued that such interventions should be directed at couples (and not individuals), as couples may have correlated weights, similar weight loss, and treatment compliance. Considering their family-building goals, both partners could also benefit from sustaining healthy behaviors across their lifespan. However, couple-based lifestyle interventions are still to be tested.

One in each five patients/couples discontinue treatment before they achieve pregnancy. Neither clinics nor patients benefit from noncompliance with treatment recommendations, but this issue does not tend to be explicitly discussed, maybe because staff fear being perceived as coercing patients into treatment. However, information on single versus cumulative pregnancy rates and on the patients' ability to undergo the repeated cycles that will maximize their chances of conceiving is important for self-care. A realistic understanding of the demands of treatment will help patients to better prepare; for instance, by conceptualizing failure as "part of the journey" or organizing in advance for multiple cycles (e.g., by revising long-term work commitments). Such approaches could also help to prevent loss of hope when confronted with failure and decisional conflict in between cycles. Knowing in advance the optimal number of cycles to maximize success may also help patients achieve "peace of mind," that they did everything in their power to facilitate long-term adjustment to failed fertility treatment[25].

Promote and Develop Tools for Shared Decision-Making

Many consider shared decision-making to be the crux of PCC, because it ensures that patients' values and preferences are fully discussed with staff and guide treatment decisions alongside evidence. A Cochrane review showed that care decided in cooperation with chronically ill patients leads to small improvements in certain psychological and physical health outcomes, as well as in patients' self-care ability[26]. Another Cochrane review showed that when clinics use decision aids, patients are more likely to discuss treatment options with their physicians, have better knowledge about their treatment options, and have better insight about what matters to them[27]. In some cases, decision aids lead to better compliance; for instance, with medication. Further, using decision aids to reach shared decisions does not worsen health outcomes nor decrease patient satisfaction.

ART patients are confronted with multiple complex decisions during their treatment process, for which they often feel ill informed (e.g., undergoing another cycle). Staff tend to assume that decisions should be made so as always to maximize patients' chances of achieving a pregnancy (and safety), but research shows that patients balance their desire for children with other valued goals; for instance, retaining emotional well-being, avoiding financial difficulties, and maintaining the partnership. Consistently, staff may be surprised to know that some patients find value in continuing treatment even when the odds to achieve a pregnancy are extremely low, because they want to achieve the "peace of mind" of knowing they tried everything they could (prevention of future regret), which is protective when treatment indeed fails[25]. These examples reveal the importance of explicitly bringing patients' values into clinical decision-making.

Unfortunately, judging by the number of decision aids targeting ART decisions, infertile patients seem to have very few opportunities to engage in shared decision-making. We are only aware of a decision aid to help patients deciding on the number of embryos to transfer in IVF. This tool, which encouraged patients to transfer a single embryo, increased patients' knowledge, had no effect on anxiety and depression, and resulted in a reduction of treatment-related costs. An area of exception seems to be oncofertility, where multiple decision aids have been developed to assist cancer patients and survivors in making fast, well-informed, and value-based decisions about whether they want to cryopreserve their fertility and how. These tools tend to be well accepted by patients and to lead to positive decision-making outcomes; for instance, lower decisional conflict and regret. Much more emphasis should be placed on the development of tools that facilitate patient–staff discussion about important diagnosis and treatment decisions.

Personalization: Adapting Care and Treatment Services to Patients

Most fertility care puts the emphasis on helping patients adapt to the demands of treatment. Personalization of treatment puts the emphasis on adapting treatment procedures to patients. For instance, most women will have to undergo hormonal stimulation. Adapting patients to treatment means informing women about the side effects of stimulation. Adapting treatment to patients implies attempting to minimize such side effects; for instance, by offering mild-stimulation or freeze-all protocols.

Personalizing care also implies putting the person and not the disease at the center of care. Within this framework, the starting point is not a clinical diagnosis but the patients' narrative of their disease within their broader life context. This implies that any treatment discussion between patients and staff needs to contemplate patients' needs and preferences not only toward care but also toward their valued position in life.

The PCC literature shows that patients value having access to comprehensive, competent, and well-organized care that minimizes time in treatment. More specifically, they value[3,13]:

- accessible treatment costs
- short travelling distances to clinics
- continuous access to clinics by phone and outside traditional nine to five working hours
- timely referrals and minimal waiting times for initiation and during treatments
- being offered and counseled regarding a comprehensive diagnosis and treatment plan
- smooth organization and coordination of diagnosis and treatment procedures among the fertility team
- being followed throughout their treatment pathway by the same physician, who also provides a good medical follow-up

Recommendations

Involve Patients in Research and Other Initiatives to Improve Quality of Care

Patients can be involved in the identification and prioritization of areas for improvement at clinics (for instance, using the PCC questionnaires listed in Table 12.2), in the design of new procedures and policies, and in the monitoring of change and its desirable (and adverse) effects. Effective patient involvement can foster mutual influence and increased agreement between patients and staff, resulting in collective decisions about changes to healthcare that will be more acceptable to patients. A cluster RCT showed that patient involvement can shift priorities in healthcare delivery to be more patient-oriented, although this collaborative process is more costly (patients' time, meal and travelling expenses) and time consuming (takes longer to reach agreement).

How can patients be involved in shaping the care they receive? Within infertility and ART, they have already successfully been involved in the identification of valued and problematic aspects of care, as well as in the evaluation of care. One study showed that it is also possible to bring staff and patients together to design clinic audits, discuss obtained results and define subsequent improvement goals[11]. Improvements observed in this study were modest, but this can be related with other factors beyond patient involvement; for instance, which improvement strategies clinics undertook once staff and patients agreed on what to improve. Another study showed that wikis (websites collaboratively developed by a community of users) are a promising way to involve patients in the co-production of information [28]. There are many examples of where patients were successfully involved in improving the feasibility and acceptability of assessment instruments, and support and decision-making tools. Patients can even be involved in advisory work to governments to influence policy change in healthcare provision, as was the case in the recent production of a report to the Welsh government about healthcare provision for endometriosis in Wales, which used the participatory method DrawingOut[21]. Finally, clinics can simply invite patients to integrate their advisory or steering groups (if they have them), which will give patients an opportunity to contribute to their clinics' strategic vision and planning. These are some promising examples of patient involvement in ART care, but there are numerous other possibilities. Table 12.2 lists available guidance for clinics interested in involving patients in their care planning and research.

Promote Patients' Positive Adjustment to Unsuccessful Fertility Treatment

Most people decide to undergo fertility treatment because they value parenthood as a central life goal. Although treatment usually involves undergoing multiple cycles during a protracted period, it represents only part of patients' life journeys in search of fulfillment and self-realization. Those patients for whom treatment is successful are likely to find meaning in life through their parenthood and caring experience. Nonetheless, the one-third of patients for whom treatment is unsuccessful will have to find other routes into a fulfilling life. It is well known that treatment success is relatively low (6 out of 10 patients will achieve a pregnancy after 3 IVF cycles; 7 out of 10 after a 5-year treatment period), difficult to predict, and affected by multiple factors beyond the control of the fertility team. A meta-analysis showed that undergoing unsuccessful treatment is associated with lower mental health and well-being (moderate effect sizes[25]). It is therefore clear clinics should put a much stronger emphasis on promoting a positive adjustment to unsuccessful treatment than they currently do.

This work should start during treatment. Indeed, patients who feel they are well advised during treatment, who receive clear explanations for why their cycles(s) fail and why their prognosis is low, who can explore all adequate treatment options, and who do not have to stop treatment due to financial issues adjust better in the aftermath of unsuccessful treatment[25]. Although both patients and staff are reluctant to discuss the possibility of failure, research shows that the capacity to imagine other future scenarios than genetic parenthood (adoption, fostering, and life without another child) facilitates adjustment during and after treatment. Interventions embedding components to foster such capacity have proved successful in promoting adjustment and self-efficacy to deal with infertility. On the contrary, focusing exclusively on achieving a pregnancy or failing to communicate realistic success rates can lead to staff difficulties in managing expectations[17] and patient feelings of abandonment and anger toward the clinic when confronted with failure[25].

The challenges patients face after treatment are very different from the ones they faced during treatment; nonetheless, so far only one intervention for the post-treatment period has been developed and evaluated. Even so, there is now significant knowledge about the psychosocial mechanisms underlying a positive adjustment to unmet parenthood goals[25]. Future research should focus on translating such knowledge into the development and testing of support interventions[13]. Meanwhile, clinics can direct their patients to charities who offer online support (see Table 12.2).

Conclusion

This review makes seven recommendations to improve the quality of PCC in ART. As stated in the introduction, it may be more feasible to work toward incremental change in PCC by addressing one recommendation at a time. How should clinics prioritize? There are three aspects to balance: the relative importance patients attribute to each PCC dimension, the evidence that changes in specific dimensions may affect desired health outcomes for patients and staff, and the specific needs of each clinic's patient population. European-level research showed that the most valued PCC dimensions are information provision and communication (engagement), as well as attitude of and relationship with staff (centeredness). Within these, information provision is clearly and consistently the most valued dimension. It is also the one most consistently associated with patient health outcomes, such as mental health and quality of life, and knowledge about and compliance with treatment. In addition, a recent review on the effect of PCC interventions on individual, relational, and social adjustment showed that information provision and psychoeducation are associated with decreases in infertility-specific stress and concerns [13]. Based on these data, our recommendation is for clinics to prioritize information provision, unless their patients have other high priority needs or preferences.

In sum, high-quality PCC should aim to respect patients and their stated preferences, needs, and values; empower patients to share the management of infertility and its treatment with the fertility treatment staff; and adapt care and treatment services to patients (instead of expecting that patients will adapt to treatments and clinics). Clinics can work toward achieving these aims by following the recommendations put forward in this chapter. It is up to clinics to prioritize change according to their patients' profiles, needs, and preferences.

Acknowledgments

I would like to thank my colleagues, Professor Jacky Boivin and Dr. Eline Dancet, for their insightful and helpful comments on a draft of this chapter.

References

1. Whelan E. Negotiating Science and Experience in Medical Knowledge: Gynaecologists on Endometriosis. *Soc Sci Med.* 2009; 68: 1489–97.

2. van Empel IWH, et al. Coming Soon to Your Clinic: High-Quality ART. *Hum Reprod.* 2008; 23: 1242–5.

3. Dancet EAF, et al. The Patients' Perspective on Fertility Care: A Systematic Review. *Hum Reprod Update* 2010; 16: 467–87.

4. Dancet EAF, et al. Patient-Centred Infertility Care: A Qualitative Study to Listen to the Patient's Voice. *Hum Reprod.* 2011; 26(4): 827–33.

5. Aarts JWM, et al. Professionals' Perceptions of Their Patients' Experiences with Fertility Care. *Hum Reprod.* 2011; 26 (5): 1119–27.

6. Aarts JWM, et al. How Patient-Centred Care Relates to Patients' Quality of Life and Distress: A Study in 427 Women Experiencing Infertility. *Hum Reprod.* 2012; 27: 488–95.

7. Gameiro S, Canavarro MC, Boivin J Patient Centred Care in Infertility Health Care: Direct and Indirect Associations with Wellbeing During Treatment. *Patient Educ Couns.* 2013; 93(3): 646–54.

8. Huppelschoten AG, et al. Predicting Dropout in Fertility Care: A Longitudinal Study on Patient-Centredness. *Hum Reprod.* 2013; 28(8): 2177–86.

9. Pedro J, et al. Positive Experiences of Patient-Centred Care Are Associated with Intentions to Comply with Fertility

Treatment: Findings from the Validation of the Portuguese Version of the PCQ-Infertility Tool. *Hum Reprod.* 2013; 28(**9**): 2462–72.

10. Dancet EA, et al. "Patient-Centered Fertility Treatment": What Is Required? *Fertil Steril.* 2014; 101(**4**): 924–6.

11. Huppelschoten AG, et al. Improving Patient-Centredness in Partnership with Female Patients: A Cluster Rct in Infertility Care. *Hum Reprod.* 2015; 30(**5**): 1137–45.

12. Garcia D, et al. Training in Empathic Skills Improves the Patient–Physician Relationship During the First Consultation in a Fertility Clinic. *Fertil Steril.* 2013; 99: 1413–18.

13. Gameiro S, et al. ESHRE Guideline: Routine Psychosocial Care in Infertility and Medically Assisted Reproduction – a Guide for Fertility Staff. *Hum Reprod.* 2015; 30(**11**): 2476–85.

14. van Empel IWH, et al. Physicians Underestimate the Importance of Patient-Centredness to Patients: A Discrete Choice Experiment in Fertility Care. *Hum Reprod.* 2011; 26(**3**): 584–93.

15. Gameiro S, et al. Why Do Patients Discontinue Fertility Treatment? A Systematic Review of Reasons and Predictors of Discontinuation in Fertility Treatment. *Hum Reprod.* 2012; 18(**6**): 652–69.

16. Benyamini Y, Gozlan M, Kokia E Variability in the Difficulties Experienced by Women Undergoing Infertility Treatments. *Fertil Steril.* 2005; 83: 275–83.

17. Boivin J, et al. Perceived Challenges of Working in a Fertility Clinic: A Qualitative Analysis of Work Stressors and Difficulties Working with Patients. *Hum Reprod.* 2017; 32(**2**): 403–8.

18. Leone D, et al. Breaking Bad News in Assisted Reproductive Technology: A Proposal for Guidelines. *Reprod Health.* 2017; 14: 87.

19. Dancet EAF, et al. Patients from Across Europe Have Similar Views on Patient-Centred Care: An International Multilingual Qualitative Study in Infertility Care. *Hum Reprod.* 2012; 27(**6**): 1702–11.

20. American Society for Reproductive Medicine. *Guidelines for advertising by ART programs.* 2004; Birmingham, AL.: American Society for Reproductive Medicine.

21. Gameiro S, et al. DrawingOut – An Innovative Drawing Workshop Method to Support the Generation and Dissemination of Research Findings. *PLoS ONE.* 2018; 13(**9**): e0203197.

22. Tarasoff LA, et al. Using Interactive Theatre to Help Fertility Providers Better Understand Sexual and Gender Minority Patients. *Medical Humanities.* 2014; **40**: 135–41.

23. Boivin J, Griffiths E, Venetis CA Emotional Distress in Infertile Women and Failure of Assisted Reproductive Technologies: Meta-Analysis of Prospective Psychosocial Studies. *BMJ.* 2011; 342(d**223**).

24. Nicoloro-SantaBarbara J, et al. Just Relax and You'll Get Pregnant? Meta-Analysis Examining Women's Emotional Distress and the Outcome of Assisted Reproductive Technology. *Soc Sci Med.* 2018; 213: 54–62.

25. Gameiro S, Finnigan A. Long-Term Adjustment to Unmet Parenthood Goals Following ART: A Systematic Review and Meta-Analysis. *Hum Reprod Update.* 2017; 23(**3**): 322–37.

26. Coulter A, et al. Personalised Care Planning for Adults with Chronic or Long-Term Health Conditions (Review). *Cochrane Library* 2015; 3: Art. No.: CD010523.

27. O'Connor AM, et al. Decision Aids for Patients Facing Health Treatment or Screening Decisions: Systematic Review. *BMJ* 1999; 319: 731.

28. van de Belt TH, et al. Wikis to Facilitate Patient Participation in Developing Information Leaflets: First Experiences. *Inform Health Soc Care.* 2014; 39(**2**): 124–39.

Chapter 13

The IVF Patient Journey of the Future

Thomas L Toth and Angela Q Leung

Since IVF led to the first successful birth over 40 years ago, it has transformed from a medical innovation focused on women with tubal occlusion to a far broader infertility and, in many instances, noninfertility therapy. The field of reproductive medicine today is nothing like what it was when it first started. As with many new technologies, the early decades were spent honing the craft, adapting laboratory and clinical innovations from animal experimentation to one that has provided a revolution in the development of complex hormonal treatments and laboratory practices (Chapters 2 and 3), including extended culture, ICSI, vitrification, and oocyte cryopreservation (Chapters 5 and 10). During that time, effort was concentrated on understanding and perfecting the technology being offered to patients. That time of great innovation led to increasing efficacy and safety of treatments, wider dissemination of information, proliferation of care, and the use of technology and integrated multidisciplinary teams to offer PCC.

While exciting clinical and technological advancements in ART are still being made today, the field is entering a new phase. Personalized treatment and the patients' experience of their journey to parenthood will be the major emphasis in coming decades. The overarching goal will be the delivery of one healthy child at a time whose adulthood will not be impacted by their parents' fertility issues or genetic risks.

As this medical field burgeons into an international community comprising medical and mental-health care providers, scientists, innovators, marketers, activists, and many more, the next 40 years will be a time of exciting growth, innovation, and transformation. The patient's experience of fertility care will be more personalized, convenient, and holistic. Seeing a fertility specialist will become a natural and routine part of the family planning process, with the ultimate goal of safely building healthy families.

An ART Cycle of the Future

We want to summarize what we envision the patient experience will look like in the not-so-distant future:

Emma is a young aspiring astronaut who dreams of being on the next shuttle into space. She is 25 years old, single, and plans to have children at a later age. During her pretraining physical and mental health assessment, the doctor reminds her of the option of FP, since Emma might be in space for an extended period with uncertain effects on her fertility. She thinks this is a great idea and asks friends on social media for clinic recommendations. She scrolls through reviews online and realizes that convenience, accessibility, and the "patient experience" are the hallmark characteristics that she is looking for.

She finds "The Fertility Center" and reviews their website. She is excited to see that all relevant information about FP and the process she would have to go through is transparent and clearly stated on the website. Although this clinic is mainly based in the metropolitan city 100 miles away, they have easy telecommunication options that make it the most convenient choice for Emma. She goes to the "New Patient" section and fills out her information on a secure online form. She immediately sees the schedule of availability for new patient appointments and picks a date and time that works for her. After registering, she receives a confirmation email and directions to download a secure app on her phone on which her profile, appointments, medical results, and treatment instructions can all be communicated. Emma is excited that this clinic is so convenient, user-friendly, and discreet, and that she does not have to rely only on telephone calls for information.

Prior to her appointment, she receives a kit to perform at-home fertility testing as deemed appropriate by her personalized fertility evaluation algorithm. The kit contains a device that plugs into her smartphone, which instantly provides laboratory results and uploads them to the clinic's app. A painless finger stick or salivary sample is all that is required for accurate testing, and the device can even perform a semen analysis. She will continue to use this device for cycle monitoring if she proceeds with egg freezing.

On the day of her appointment, Emma logs into her smartphone app to attend the teleconference appointment with her fertility team. She meets her doctor as well as the administrative assistant, nurse, financial counselor, and wellness coach. The fertility panel test results, which were completed prior to her appointment, are available for review and, as a team, they discuss her fertility goals and options. Using an AI-generated algorithm, her history and initial tests help formulate a personalized treatment plan to optimize her chance of success. Her treatment plan includes not only the medical aspects necessary to achieve her egg freezing goal but also nutrition, exercise, and mental-health counseling to promote overall wellness. By the end of the appointment, Emma has a clear understanding of her next steps with written instructions on how to proceed outlined in her app.

Emma follows her personalized treatment algorithm, which continually provides the best personalized pathway, protocol, and medication dosing for her cycle. Prior to starting, her financial counselor discusses the best strategy to optimize her financial resources. She also receives teleconference teaching on how and when to take the cycle medications and how to perform home monitoring. These videos are recorded and stored in her app, which she can refer to anytime she has questions. Emma is so thankful that the stimulation medications are oral; she had heard that, in the past, patients had to give themselves injections. Emma is sent a home ultrasound monitoring device and instructed on how to use it properly. On the days when she is instructed via the app to do monitoring, she performs a home ultrasound and her follicle growth data is uploaded directly to her chart in the electronic medical record. She also performs a finger stick blood test at home with the smartphone device that analyzes a droplet of blood. All hormone testing is remote, and her ultrasound and bloodwork results are uploaded via the app directly to the clinic. Based on her results, she receives a text via the app from her care team who give her instructions regarding her medications. Emma finds this system extremely easy and convenient to navigate, especially given that the clinic's physical location is so far away. In the past, patients had to travel almost every day during their cycle to a clinic site for traditional phlebotomy and ultrasound. Emma cannot imagine the inconvenience and cost this would incur to many people – no wonder so few people accessed fertility services in the past. Nowadays, almost everyone Emma knows has had at least a consultation regarding fertility planning. An increasingly broader range of couples and single people are routinely utilizing fertility services with improved accessibility of reproductive clinics in the United States and the world.

The day of her egg retrieval arrives and is performed at a convenient clinic location of her choosing. The process is painless and no longer requires traditional anesthesia, as it had in the past. Advances in other fields of medicine also aid fertility treatment and newly developed oral medication allows the retrieval procedure to be performed painlessly. As part of her holistic wellness care, she also receives acupuncture and massage services that day to help alleviate stress.

Her gametes are processed using specific tagging systems linked to Emma's personal identification data. The eggs that are retrieved are processed by an embryologist using a microfluidic device, which prepares the eggs for fertilization or freezing. In Emma's case, her eggs are cryopreserved by the automated system and transferred to a secure storage facility where they will remain until Emma has need of them. All her eggs have a specific tag, which links them to her patient profile and tracks their location, temperature, and gas parameters in the lab, thus ensuring identification. Via this electronic tagging, Emma is also able to track her eggs herself on her smartphone app, which provides her reassurance that they are safe. All data are maintained using block chain technology, which allows her to access information from any location.

Ten years later, Emma has met the love of her life, Liam, and they are ready to start building a family. Incidentally, Liam also froze his sperm at a younger age when his personalized genetic risk assessment determined a high risk of testicular cancer. Together, they return to the clinic where Emma had her eggs frozen to discuss their options for conception. Even though they now live in the city where the clinic is located, they continue to use the teleconferencing option as it is more convenient for their busy schedules. However, Emma has heard from her friends who have visited the clinic that it does not look like a traditional doctor's office at all, but more like a nice salon or spa. Many clinics are recognizing that patients often do not want to be in an overly medicalized setting, which has led to the delinking of fertility centers from hospital settings, and a change in the aesthetic of the physical spaces. This makes the entire process more comfortable and feel more "natural," especially since family planning is such an integral part of many people's lives.

Emma and Liam undergo home fertility testing using a similar device Emma had used when freezing her eggs. However, this time, no blood or saliva sample is even needed – the device simply scans their skin to produce instantaneous results. They are amazed at how far technology has advanced in 10 short years. After meeting with their fertility team – the same team that helped Emma many years ago – they are ready to tackle the next steps as outlined by their personalized treatment algorithm. They opt to use their frozen gametes to create embryos for transfer.

While waiting for her treatment to begin, Emma and Liam feel increasingly anxious about their ability to conceive and upcoming treatment. Their team checks in at regular intervals and discusses their desires, goals, and fears, and how they may impact the treatment. Their wellness coach also shows them both physical and mental exercises to perform to help with anxiety. They appreciate that now there is an increased understanding among medical professionals that the mind and body are intricately linked and, especially in stressful situations such as family building, the care of the whole person is paramount. Many more clinics now employ or partner with psychologists, social workers, nutritionists, acupuncturists, and massage therapists. Mental health and wellness are an integral part of fertility care. Emma and Liam feel grateful for the empathy shown by the clinic staff, as well as the personalized and integrated care they have received. With the support of their team, they feel ready to tackle the next steps.

Emma's frozen eggs and Liam's frozen sperm are retrieved from the robotic storage facility and are processed using an automated device that selects the most viable sperm for insemination. The process of fertilization, embryo culture, and embryo assessment are performed within an automated microfluidic platform, which eliminates environmental exposure and human error. All the embryos have a specific tag, which allows Emma and Liam to track the progress of the embryos. This provides them reassurance and also helps them feel connected to the growth of their early embryos. Noninvasive preimplantation genetic and viability marker testing is performed and, while results are pending, the embryos are cryopreserved in an automated machine that stores the embryos. The genetic testing that is performed can comprehensively examine the genome for each embryo and determine the highest implantation potential and healthiest offspring. In combination with the metabolic and morphologic data collected through time-lapse imaging, an AI program amasses and analyzes all the data to rank the embryos for transfer.

Based on Emma's testing, her personalized treatment algorithm has determined the optimal receptive day for an ET. A single embryo is retrieved according to its ranked viability potential from the automated system and thawed. The transfer goes well and, while Emma is enduring the difficult wait for her pregnancy test, her team has planned a regimen to assist with healthy dietary choices, and physical and mental exercises. Happily, Emma finds out that she is pregnant! After her confirmatory first trimester ultrasound, she is introduced to an obstetrician who works closely with her fertility team. Throughout her pregnancy, she continues to receive wellness support, including nutrition and exercise counseling, mental health exercises, and parenting classes. Emma also joins an online support community and shares her journey with fertility treatment with others. She eventually delivers a healthy newborn.

Emma and Liam truly feel that their success was a team effort, spearheaded by people who cared about both their physical and emotional journey through family building.

They feel confident that they can reach their goal of three children with the help of their team. In fact, Emma plans to refer her single younger sister to them to discuss her desires about future fertility. After all, fertility care is not just about treating people who have difficulty conceiving – it is about providing the framework for family building so that it is a natural and routine part of a lifelong journey.

Index